Tactical Barbe

AGELESS ATHLETE

Jim Madden, PhD

ISBN-13: 978-1544080826
ISBN-10: 1544080824

Consult a physician before beginning this program or any new fitness regime.

Thanks to K.B. The best guy I never met.

CONTENTS

PART 1:
POSSIBILITIES

Those who devote themselves exclusively to physical training turn out to be more savage than they should, while those who devote themselves to music and poetry turn out to be softer than is good for them.

Plato, Republic[1]

CHAPTER 1:
TEN YEARS TO MULTIDIMENSIONAL FITNESS

I turned thirty in 2003 with a tremendous sense of satisfaction on that birthday. I had a great marriage (and thankfully I still do), a healthy son, and a good start on my career as a professor of philosophy. I felt like I had finally arrived somewhere as a *bona fide* husband, father, and professional. My twenties had been a whirlwind: college, graduate school, and moving around the United States as my wife and I started our careers. In the end, it had all worked out, and we had landed firmly on the ground. Suffice it to say, I had much to be happy about at the close of my third decade on earth.

There was, nevertheless, an eight-hundred-pound gorilla I had been ignoring. In fact, you could say that it was more like a three-hundred-pound gorilla, and the ape was me! I stand only 5'8", but at the time I probably weighed over three hundred pounds. I'm sure that I don't need to inform anyone that, whatever you think of the standard BMI scale, that height-to-weight ratio is bad news. I say "probably three hundred pounds" because I just didn't have the guts to step on a scale and face the humiliating truth. I could dodge the scale, but I could not ignore the mirror: I had arrived at my thirtieth birthday very fat. I resolved at that point in my life to change that fact. With the really important things (family and career) progressing with good momentum, it was time for me to work on the obvious problem I had been ignoring. My self-imposed ignorance had to end.

Up to a certain point, it was actually pretty easy to deceive myself about my obesity. Like a lot of American kids, I started playing organized sports when I was in primary school with baseball and basketball. I struggled at those sorts of sports (and I still can't make a basket to save my life). All that changed when in middle school I was introduced to football and wrestling, which rewarded brute strength. The summer before seventh grade I started lifting weights, and by the time I was a freshman in high school I weighed 200lbs and could bench press 275lbs. Brute strength and size were reaping great dividends for me both on the field and socially. I started to identify myself as "a big strong guy." As I mentioned above, I'm pretty short, but I did go on to play NCAA Division III college football. I kept getting bigger and stronger, and at that level I did pretty well (I started for three seasons and was captain of my team). By the time I finished playing in college I was a solid 250-pound fireplug.

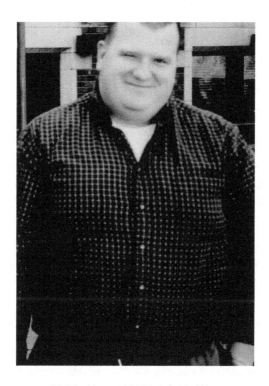

Jim Madden on his thirtieth birthday.

Football gave me a lot, but it also took a lot from me. I suppose that is true for most guys who play that sport. It was fun, but by the time I was twenty-two years old I was an orthopedic mess. I had multiple stress fractures in my fifth lumbar vertebrae that gave me a lot pain, and I generally felt like an old man. When I finished playing, I never wanted to do another "gasser" again, and I went off to graduate school with single-minded determination for my field of study. That is all well and good, but when you are used to eating (and drinking beer!) like a guy who pumps iron every morning and then runs wind sprints and knocks heads at practice every night, the pounds will really pack on in a hurry when those activities cease. I didn't really notice. I was "a big strong guy," right? I had been rewarded for getting ever bigger for my entire adolescence and early adulthood. Without knowing it (or at least admitting it), "the big strong guy" was becoming "the big fat guy."

I competed in powerlifting in high school, and about midway through my Ph.D. studies I took up the sport again. This was not because I felt the need to get into shape. I just missed competition, and the only sort of sport I could envision myself excelling in was something that rewarded brute strength. I remember telling someone at that time that "I compete in powerlifting because I'm only good at sports that involve picking up heavy objects or colliding with other men who are good at picking up heavy objects." I wasn't world class, but I got pretty strong using mainly Westside Barbell methods. In competition, I squatted 660lbs and bench pressed 425lbs. In the gym I hit 700lbs and 450 respectively. My deadlift really struggled relative to those lifts, 550lbs. (More on that below.) As my life got more demanding with the transition from graduate school and the arrival of our first baby, powerlifting got put on the back-burner.

Naturally when I decided on my thirtieth birthday that it was time to address my obesity, I saw the problem through the lens of my prior training experience. I had been training for fifteen years almost entirely to get bigger and stronger. Strength and mass were my prime ends. Certainly, playing football required conditioning—lots of it. Notice, however, that my conditioning for football was almost entirely sprinting and high intensity calisthenics (think lots of burpees). We did almost nothing in the way of classic aerobic conditioning. In fact, linemen like me were mostly told to avoid distance running because that sort of thing supposedly would make you skinny and weak. I remember my senior year in college trying to go out for a two-mile jog and nearly dying! As a short offensive lineman, my strength was my only advantage, so that was my prime focus. Conditioning was a box that had to be checked (minimally) but only through a single modality (sprinting). When I took up powerlifting, I doubled-down on this emphasis.

Thus, for me "getting back into shape" meant a return to max effort good mornings, twenty-rep squat cycles, and the like. My conditioning approach was exclusively sprints, and even that was done too sparingly. I made some progress, but sooner or later my back always gave out or I would pull a hamstring, which would put me out of commission for six weeks. Everything was "one step forward, two steps back." The obvious problem was that I had a one-dimensional approach to fitness. **I mistook being fit with simply being strong.** Moreover, I had identified myself as being a big strong guy, so the idea of having to give that up was psychologically untenable. I was operating with bad "either/or" thinking: I thought that I had to decide between being *either* weak and pathetic *or* a breathy powerlifter. This myopic approach was not only preventing me from making progress but had me stuck on a vicious treadmill of injury and frustration. I was just too heavy, and I lacked the background endurance capacity to push hard in my anaerobic conditioning without burnout and injury.

Things changed in 2006 when I discovered kettlebells. The game-changer was not the kettlebell *per se*. There are advantages to that tool (I love them and I have been using them in my training for ten years now), but there is no deep magic emanating from a cannonball with a handle. The key ingredient for me was the style of programing typically associated with kettlebells. Take, for example, Pavel Tsatsouline's programs.[2]

You get a recommendation to do short, heavy, high frequency strength training sessions, with a mind to gaining strength without mass while optimizing recovery. Conditioning is likewise done in smaller and frequent bursts designed to get results while leaving a lot in your tank for other activities.

After playing around with kettlebells mostly haphazardly for a few months, I set to work on achieving Pavel's Rite of Passage standards: 200 hundred snatches with a 24KG kettlebell in ten minutes and pressing "The Beast" (48KG kettlebell). I made sensible dietary changes; as I put it now, I quit eating like I had a death wish. I also started doing some light jogging on my off days to help with my lungs for the grueling snatches. By the summer of 2007 I had swung, snatched, pressed, and jogged my way to passing the Rite of Passage and losing over eighty pounds along the way. For the first time since I was a teenager, I weighed less than 220lbs. A year earlier I would not have thought that possible. Moreover, for the first time in over a decade injury and pain were not a regular part of my life because of problems I was having in my training.

The thing to notice for our purposes is that I had, almost accidently, gone from being a one-trick pony (a pure strength athlete) to a multidimensional athlete, i.e., someone building capabilities in aerobic endurance (jogging), anaerobic work capacity (swinging and snatching kettlebells), and max strength (cleaning and pressing kettle-bells) simultaneously. The effect on my body composition and athletic performance was tremendous. That year of training revealed to me possibilities I would not have previously imagined. Training to improve my performance across multiple fitness domains was the big game-changer for me.

At that point I vowed never to go back, and thus far I have not waivered. I began to approach fitness with both the athletic and the scholarly skills I had built through my education. I began to read voraciously on topics in exercise and fitness. I experimented with various programs and exercises. I continued to compete in powerlifting occasionally, but as the years went on I moved further from a pure strength mentality and toward a sophisticated multi-dimensional approach.

Fast forward seven years to to my fortieth birthday in 2013. I completed a tough 5K trail race in about 21 minutes. I weighed 188lbs (the lightest I had been since eighth grade!), but earlier that week I had deadlifted 500x3 casually. The prior summer I ran a 5:56 mile, just as I had done twenty dead-hang pull-ups for the first time in my life. The following spring, I would go on to bench press 350lbs, squat 500lbs, and deadlift 600lbs while maintaining a bodyweight in the 190s. I have since run half-marathons, easily swum 1600 meters, and competed in triathlons and Brazilian jiu-jitsu, while still maintaining similar strength numbers. In short, I have become a multidimensional athlete. As of this writing I am forty-three years old and am in the best overall shape of my entire life.

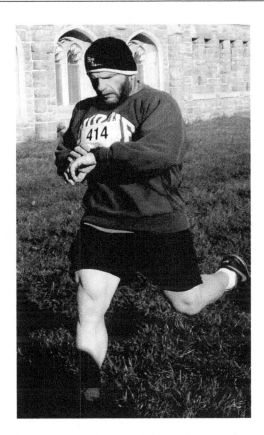

Jim Madden in 2013 on his fortieth birthday.

I'm telling you this to give you a concrete example of what the possibilities really are. **I'm nobody special. What I am going to outline in the rest of this book is within your grasp.** My journey has shown me that a smart, multi-dimensional fitness program is the key to sustained high performance over the course of a lifetime. **If I can do it and reap these sorts of results, then so can you.**

My transformation transpired entirely in my thirties and forties, the period of our lives in which we have all been conditioned to begin to expect physical decline. I don't claim to have the fountain of youth—far from it. Nevertheless, I hope this book will show that there are readily available pathways that will help you kick that can down the road into the indefinite future. If you are already middle-aged, then let's discuss how you can address the issues you are likely facing. If you are younger, then let me suggest to you a line of thought that will set you on a course for decades of fitness.

The following chapters are not based on any scientific studies that I have personally conducted. I am not that kind of doctor! This is a book about my experience as a multi-dimensional athlete. Though not necessarily scientifically verified, everything in this book is battle-tested either by me or people I have trained over the years. These are the methods and ideas that I have developed throughout three decades of training. Help yourself to disagree. That's great: I'm in the disagreement business. Probably, however, you will find that these principles and programs are readily applicable to your own training.

You will see me refer to K. Black's *Tactical Barbell* and *Tactical Barbell II: Conditioning*[3] throughout this text. When I encountered K. Black's work I found a tightly organized, systematic presentation of the hodgepodge of ideas I had conglomerated from various authors and my own experiences over the years. I had been following something akin to Tactical Barbell for years without knowing it. I now structure almost all of my training according to the parameters of the Tactical Barbell system. You don't need to have these books in front of you to implement everything I am going to recommend; you could substitute whatever equivalent strength and conditioning programs you have in your toolbox. Nevertheless, Tactical Barbell is the best system I am aware of, and in what follows we will apply it to questions of lifelong fitness.

CENTRAL TAKE-AWAYS FROM CHAPTER 1

- **Radical physical transformation is a possible**, even after decades of inveterate bad habits and confused thinking.

- **A multi-dimensional approach to fitness** is both an effective and sustainable means to such a transformation.

- The **Tactical Barbell system** provides a reliable platform to multi-dimensional fitness.

CHAPTER 2:
PSYCHOLOGICAL PITFALLS

QUIT SAYING "I KNOW THAT SINCE I'M FORTY, I CAN'T..."

You are probably thinking that this is a book for the *middle-aged athlete* or the *older trainee.* Maybe you are thinking that this is a book for the "over forty crowd." In light of both its title and my remarks in the last chapter, I understand how you could get that impression. Fair enough, but let's get something clear at the beginning: this is no such book. In fact, **I don't believe there should be such books!**

Certainly, some explanation is in order. Sports psychologists caution athletes against thinking about what they don't want to do instead of what they want to do. David Mack and Gary Casstevens make the point using the example of a golfer trying to negotiate a water hazard:

> What we've learned in psychology is that actions follow our thoughts and images. If you say "Don't hit it in the water," and you're looking at the water, you have just programmed your mind to send the ball to a watery grave. The law of dominant thought says your mind is going to remember the most dominant thought. Think water, remember water, and water likely is what you will get.
>
> Rather than say "Don't hit it in the water," try another instruction, like "Land the ball ten yards to the right of the pin." You get what your mind sets. The mind works most effectively when you're telling it what to do rather than what not to do.[4]

The point is that what we consciously dwell on amounts to a sort of mental dress rehearsal for our actual actions. As any high school football coach or music teacher will tell you, "You practice like you play," and the same goes for whether you are physically or mentally practicing. That is the **Law of Dominant Thoughts**. You will act out what you think. On the one hand, if you focus on what you wish to avoid, you are practicing failure. Try it sometime. Think about *not doing something*. What is your mental picture? It is probably an image of the very activity you are thinking of not doing. When you think about not doing something, you are focusing on an image of your failure. On the other hand, if you focus on what you wish to achieve, you are practicing success. Try the opposite of our thought experiment, and think this time about something you want to do. Once again, what is your mental image? I bet it is exactly the task you want to pull off. You are mentally practicing for success.

Don't mistake this point for pie-in-the-sky positive thinking. No one here, anyway, is suggesting that to do well you should delude yourself with unwarranted optimism. The point is not that positive thinking ("I think I can, I know I can...") is actually going to make you successful. Rather, the point is that you need to conceptualize your actions in terms of what you want them to achieve, not in terms of failures you are trying to avoid. You need to suggest to yourself actual courses of action that take you to your goals, instead of ill-defined omens of failure. Your body can only follow where your mind's eye gazes, so you need to point it where you want to go.

This point really helped me with my deadlift. For years I struggled with leaning too far forward at the initiation of the movement. I constantly cued myself with "Don't lean forward." It never worked. The same painful pattern always returned whenever the loads got heavy. As soon as I started cueing myself with "Keep your shoulders behind the bar," the problem mostly corrected. I went from focusing on failure to focusing on what I had to do to achieve success, and that made all the difference. It is very hard to make yourself *not do* something (maybe impossible), so you need to make yourself *actually do* something.

Almost every semester I have conversations with students who are obsessing over what will happen if they fail one of my examinations. They always want to know whether there will be extra credit or how well they will have to do on the term paper to raise their grades. What does the Law of Dominant Thought tell you about these students? They are planning for failure, so they are contributing to their failure. I always tell them to quit thinking about failing the examination and to start thinking about what you can do to ace it. Sometimes they even listen to this advice.

Consider not only how you think about particular movements, skills, examinations, etc., but the way you conceptualize a large-scale project. Suppose you are going off to college, but you think of your education solely in terms of not flunking out. Does that actually suggest any positive action to take you toward your degree? No. You are defining your education in terms of a failure. Where is your focus? Failure. What does the Law of Dominant Thought suggest that will get you? Failure. Suppose now you define your education in terms of a certain career path, a definite goal of graduating with honors, or admission to a prestigious graduate program. Does that sort of thinking suggest an actual course of action leading to positive results? Yes. What is the object of your focus? The actions that will get you the kind of education you want. That's how you make the Law of Dominant Thought work for you on a larger scale.

The same idea holds for your fitness program. Suppose you define your program primarily in terms of avoiding failure? "This time I'm not going to skip workouts!" "I'm not going to cheat on my diet!" What is dominating your thinking? Your imagined failures. What will the Law of Dominant Thought deliver in that case? Failure. Instead, what do you get if you think of your program in terms like this? "This time I'm going to get my workouts done before work so I won't miss them when I'm on overtime," or, "I'm going to eat 1 gram of protein per pound of bodyweight." In this case you are thinking about what makes for success, so you are on the upside of the Law of Dominant Thought. Moreover because you are thinking about where you want to go, you are recommending to yourself specific actions aimed at getting there.

I answer a lot of questions on the tacticalbarbell.com forum from middle-aged trainees and trainees nervously approaching that stage of life. I have also advised a lot of friends and colleagues who want to "get back into shape" now that they have reached "a certain age." A clear pattern in their thinking has emerged. Suppose Smitty is a typical trainee of this sort. Nine out of ten times Smitty starts the conversation with something like this:

"SINCE I'M NOW IN MY FORTIES, I KNOW I CAN'T..."

Smitty completes this sentence with "run an 18 min 5K," "bench 300," "get really good body composition," or what have you. However Smitty fills in the blank, he has defined his project by his perceived limitations. What is his dominant thought? It's what he thinks he can't do. What will the Law of Dominant Thought deliver for Smitty? It will satisfy his prediction of failure. Because of this psychological mechanism, Smitty has begun his fitness project with a self-fulfilling prophecy predicting his own limitations. So the first problem is that Smitty's very way of conceptualizing his project at the beginning has imposed a limitation on what he is likely to achieve. Smitty would do better by starting with the thought of what he is going to do: "I'm going to run a sub-21 min 5K" or "I'm going to bench 275," etc. Even if he sets his goals a bit lower, he has begun the project on positive footing, and the Law of Dominant Thought is likely to reward that sound first step.

There is a deeper problem with Smitty's thinking. Why is he so quick to accept these diminished goals? Who says the forty-year-old Smitty can't run that 18 min 5K? Bench press 300? See his abs? There are people a lot older who meet and exceed these goals. We live in a youth-obsessed culture that wants us to believe that as soon as you reach your thirtieth birthday you can expect only a continuous and steep physical decline. Certainly, if you look around you will see plenty of middle-aged people in horrible condition, but who says it must be that way? Look at pictures from the nineteenth and early twentieth centuries. Do you see many people in those photographs, even in their forties, fifties, and sixties in terrible shape? Search the internet. You will find dozens of very high-achieving athletes, well into middle age and far beyond. High levels of fitness are achievable well into middle age and far beyond.

I'm sure most of you reading this are familiar with fitness author and television host Jack Lalanne, who maintained incredible levels of multidimensional fitness into his nineties. Just consider the following feats Lalanne managed during his supposedly declining years:

- Lalanne set a world push-up record at forty-two, surpassing a thousand in just twenty-three minutes

- When Lalanne was forty-five he did a thousand jumping jacks and a thousand pull-ups in one hour and twenty-two minutes

- On his seventieth birthday Lalanne completed a 1.5 mile swim in the Pacific Ocean

That is just to name a few of Lalanne's incredible physical feats, and not surprisingly the guy also maintained an impressive physique and vital lifestyle for his entire (long!) life.[5]

Though I could never endorse his love for skin-tight shiny jumpsuits, I see Lalanne as an exemplar for lifelong fitness. Thinking of guys like Lalanne, I have to snicker a bit every time I read a post on some fitness forum that begins with "I'm turning *thirty* soon, so I know I need to cut back." Seriously? There are guys in their mid-forties very effectively fighting in pro-MMA bouts, people in their seventies running ultra-marathons, and powerlifters moving huge loads in their fifties. **By accepting this unfounded, youth-obsessed foolishness, you are defeating yourself before you even try to find your real limits.** Just to drive this point home, I will periodically profile high-performing ageless athletes throughout this book. Prepare to be humbled and inspired.

I am not saying we won't decline. We are all on a (hopefully) slow one-way ticket toward physical diminishment and ultimately the grave. Remember, I'm a philosophy professor, so I spend every day of my professional life thinking and talking about the riddles of life and death. Plato famously defined philosophy as "practice for dying." Nevertheless, the fact of our mortality doesn't tell us how much of our diminishment is self-imposed, nor does it tell us how much of it we can forestall. At the very least, we don't need to give in without a fight. The fact that I will one day fade doesn't change the fact that right now in my mid-forties I feel better and am more physically capable than I have ever been.

That is why I don't think we should be writing books for the "older trainee" or the "middle-aged" athlete. Those monikers assume limitations upfront. They operate under the assumption that we can immediately expect less now that we have reached a certain age. Such an approach is the height of defining our actions by our perceived (and mostly self-imposed) limitations, and we know what the Law of Dominant

Thought delivers in such cases. If that is how we think about our fitness projects, then just like our hypothetical Smitty we have begun by predicting our own failure, which of course will contribute to our actual failure.

Instead, I am writing this book for **Ageless Athletes**. That is for people who are serious about a lifetime of high performance. There are two important concepts implied by term "lifetime." First, it invokes **continuity** between youth and middle-age. There is no hard line, and everyone is going to have a different experience with this transition. Our goal is to extend high-level performance indefinitely into the future—for a lifetime. Your capacities certainly will fade, but when and to what extent are variables you can do much to control. You are ageless not in the sense that you are exempt from the human condition, but in the sense that you won't allowed your age needlessly to foreclose the possibilities of achievement. Our thinking is focused not on accepting self-imposed limitations, but on how to maintain (or progress!) high-fitness performance into an indefinite future.

Second, "lifetime" also invokes **patience**. Notice that ten years elapsed between the two pictures of me that appear in chapter 1. That span of time is very important to emphasize. My results came after a decade of trial and error, day-in day-out dedication to exercise and diet, setbacks and false starts, and the occasional jump forward. This didn't happen to me overnight, and what really made the difference were very small steps that accumulated over the years. Radical progress might happen for you more quickly, but it will take time. It is essential that you start to think of your fitness progress not in terms of weeks or months, but in terms of years and maybe even decades. Being in a hurry is what leads to discouragement, injury, and frustration. Your question should not be "Where will I be next month." Rather, you need to **start thinking about where you will be a decade from now**. A recurring theme of this book will be the virtues of **patience** and dogged **discipline** as keys to long-term progress. Stop distorting your thoughts with the false promises of "12 Weeks to Elite Fitness" sham programs. That kind of impatience is for kids. You are a mature adult who is about to take up a patient and disciplined approach aimed at results that last a lifetime.

THE SAME LAWS OF PHYSICS APPLY TO YOU!

I want to introduce two phenomena that have been well documented by social psychologists. The first is usually called **fundamental attribution error**.[6] Suppose Smitty is driving down the road when he is passed by another car flying along at 20mph over the speed limit. What social psychologists have found is that Smitty is overwhelmingly likely to account for the other driver's behavior by attributing to him an *internal* state or disposition. For example, Smitty will say "That guy is driving that way because *he is reckless*" or "He must *think he is immune* to the law." It is the other guy's character that leads him to misbehave. Likewise, suppose Smitty loses out in competition for promotion to his colleague Jones. Smitty is likely to attribute significant powers and talents to Jones: "Who could beat Jones? He has a degree from

Columbia, and the guy is always the smartest person in the room!" Maybe less chari-tably Smitty says, "I knew Jones would get the promotion! He spends his whole day kiss'n up to the boss." Once again, the other guy gets ahead (for good or ill) by factors internal to him. The point is that when explaining other people's behavior (either successes or failures), we tend to do so by attributing to them intrinsic talents and traits of character.

On the other side of the coin, social psychologists have documented a **self-serving bias**.[7] Suppose that it is now Smitty who finds himself driving recklessly. He will explain his own behavior not by attributing to himself a state of character (recklessness), but by appealing to some sort of external circumstance: "I wouldn't drive so fast if it weren't for my boss's unreasonable demand that I get to work early today." Likewise, when asked to explain why he didn't get the promotion (as opposed to why Jones did), Smitty is likely to say something to the effect of "I would've got the nod, if it weren't for all the demands of my family life." That is, we tend to interpret our own failings in terms of external factors beyond our control. It's not my fault! There is always something outside of us that explains our shortcomings. However, supposing Smitty got the promotion, then he is likely to interpret his success internally: "This reflects my talents and my work ethic." We account for our successes, not surpris-ingly, through our own doings or good traits.

So here is the point, and this should be no surprise to anyone who has dealt with human beings in their natural environment. **We tend to interpret reality in ways that put us in a favorable light in comparison to other people**. On the one hand, when other people do better than we do, we attribute that to their unparalleled natural talents, cheating, unfair advantages, or external circumstances that hampered our own performance. On the other hand, when we are successful, we tend to see the outcome solely in terms our own efforts and talents, while we ignore external factors that gave us advantages. **The human psyche has a built in self-aggrandizing and excuse-making mechanism that skews our self-assessments**. As my high school football coach often said, "Excuses are like assholes. Everyone has one."

Anyone concerned with performance—in any of life's arenas—should be wary of this tendency. Without critical reflection, we are likely to miss why it is that we have or have not been successful. Our tendencies to celebrate our victories and excuse our defeats can blind us from understanding how we come to those ends. If we don't know the real causes of our situation and instead believe our own convenient self-serving biases, we will be unable to reproduce or avoid such outcomes in the future.

If you have spent time advising people on their fitness, then you have heard Smitty say something like this:

> "I can't get to the same level as that guy; he is clearly genetically gifted."

> "There's no way I can get in seriously good shape when I have so many family and professional demands."

"Maybe I could do that, if I were twenty-two years old like her and willing to take steroids."

Do those remarks sound familiar? Many people, especially among the "untrained," think of very fit people as extreme genetic outliers or cheaters. They are demigods and superheroes who have incredible natural gifts that open possibilities unavailable to mere mortals. Less charitably, there is also a quick rush to attribute the use of performance-enhancing drugs or a pathologically unbalanced lifestyle to everyone who is successful athletically. Likewise, our own fitness shortcomings are usually attributed to our age, professional and family demands, or whatever other excuse our self-serving bias mechanism can muster.

I don't deny that there are genetic outliers and natural advantages/disadvantages. Not everyone is going to achieve physically what is done by NFL linebackers, people on the podium at the Ironman, or Delta Force operators. There is no way I'm going to play in the NBA. We all have natural limitations. I also don't deny that some people's incredible progress has much to do with a willingness to take drugs and to go to risky extremes that many of us wisely avoid. Certainly.

Nevertheless, ask yourself this: when I look at another athlete and say "I can't do that because..." **is that conclusion a reasonable assessment of my possibilities or just one more self-serving delusion spit out by my excuse-making mechanism?** Ordinary, non-drug using, dedicated parents and professionals do in fact reach very high levels of athletic achievement. Bear that in mind the next time you are about to fall prey to your own self-serving biases. I say this to help you see that many of our limitations are really self-imposed. They are convenient biases that preserve comfortable self-conceptions. The sooner we free ourselves from these self-serving biases, the sooner we can set on a path to real achievement.

When you see very fit people you are looking at individuals who have deftly exploited the laws of physics to their advantage: force against resistance to produce adaptations, calories consumed vs. calories burned, etc. They aren't miracles. It's just the operation of the basic physical principles running the universe in conjunction with years of consistent training and nutrition. **Whatever their circumstances in comparison to yours, those same laws of physics govern your body, too.** There is no reason to think that you can't get a long way down their same path, whatever your own internal voices tell you, if you are consistent in fitness practices. Begin by taking successful ageless athletes not as markers of your limitations but as exemplars of what you can achieve.

CENTRAL TAKE-AWAYS FROM CHAPTER 2

- The **Law of Dominant Thought**: You will do as you think, so concentrate on positive steps toward success, not limitations and failure. If you define your training in terms of what you can't do at your stage of life, then you will only live up to those diminished expectations.

- The notion of "the middle-aged trainee" is a prediction of failure or limitation. Rather, think of your fitness in terms of being an **ageless athlete**: someone dedicated to the virtues of **patience** and **discipline** resulting in **continuous, high-level performance for a lifetime**.

- The human mind has a tendency to skew our interpretations in favor of excuses and self-aggrandizement. This tendency can easily lead us to set unnecessary limitations on our performance. Start by considering how these self-serving biases might be hampering your own ability to assess the real possibilities open to you. Is your claim that you are too old or too busy to achieve a high level of fitness a **self-serving bias**?

AGELESS ATHLETE PROFILE
DON WILDMAN

Don Wildman is an octogenarian and founder of Bally's Total Fitness. A Korean War combat veteran, Wildman also has a long resume of extreme athletic achievements including nine Ironman Triathlons, multiple big league marathons, and the grueling Race Across America 3,000-mile cycling race, just to name a few. Even today his regime is nearly unparalleled. He performs an infamous weight and calisthenic circuit three days a week that tallies to over three thousand nearly non-stop repetitions over a two-hour duration. He rides his bike for dozens of miles every day, paddle boards three days each week, and he also surfs and does helicopter snowboarding. Wildman is unstoppable even in his eighties! I don't know about you, but reading about Wildman robbed me of a lot of my silly excuses.[8]

PART 2:
WHY YOU SHOULD TRAIN LIKE AN OPERATIONAL ATHLETE

Now there are short and simple exercises which tire the body rapidly, and so save our time; and time is something of which we ought to keep strict account. These exercises are running, brandishing weights, and jumping.... Select for practice any one of these, and you will find it plain and easy. But whatever you do, come back soon from body to mind.

Seneca, *Moral Epistles*[9]

CHAPTER 3:
ACHIEVING BALANCE BY MODERATION

THE OPERATIONAL ATHLETE'S PUZZLE

I am not a tactical professional. I have never served in the armed forces, nor have I ever worked in law enforcement or public safety in any way. I am a desk jockey academic all the way down, and I am thankful for all of you who do real jobs that give me the leisure to sit around and read books all day. I also have a very low tolerance for the "tacticool" fitness trend. I loathe products aimed at civilians with titles like "Warrior Fitness" or "Train like a SEAL." If you want to find out what it is like to be a warrior, there are several active "government programs" that would be happy to let you try out the real thing!

Nevertheless, as I developed my own training approach I increasingly found myself gravitating toward programs produced by and aimed at tactical professionals. The attraction wasn't the illusion that I could match mettle with an Army Ranger by achieving a certain time in a 10K. Hardly! I'm a wimp about getting enough sleep, and I've never really enjoyed camping. Rather, it always seemed obvious to me that many tactical professionals are in incredibly good physical condition, so it stood to reason to look into what they were doing. It was that curiosity that led me to pick up a copy of *Tactical Barbell*.

I had studied and experimented with a several programs aimed at tactical and rescue professionals over the years, but it was *Tactical Barbell* and *Tactical Barbell II* that really resonated with the intuitions about training that I had developed, especially with what I was learning about what worked best for me as I entered my forties. In this and the following chapter I want to outline why I came to the conclusion that **the Tactical Barbell system is ideal for the ageless athlete**. This discussion will also serve as a review of the key concepts of the Tactical Barbell system that are presupposed by the later parts of this book.

The Tactical Barbell system is a comprehensive strength and conditioning program designed to serve police, rescue, and military professionals. The central concept of the system is the notion of an **Operational Athlete**, which K. Black defines as follows: "an individual required to (a) **excel** in (b) **multiple fitness domains** (c) **simultaneously** – (d) **at any given time**." Let's take the time to analyze the components of this definition in detail.[10]

(A) EXCEL

The operational athlete needs to have better than average levels of fitness, and for most tactical professions that means far better than average. The operational athlete may not be elite in any one fitness attribute, e.g., he is probably not going to bench press 500lbs, but he or she needs to possess multiple advanced or superior attributes, e.g., the ability to bench press 350lbs pounds while also being able to run 5K in <20 min, and perform 20 pull-ups. Of course pulling off *all* of those feats is itself an elite achievement! Nobody is recommending mediocrity—just a different kind of excellence suited to a particular sort of work.

(B) MULTIPLE FITNESS DOMAINS

As implied above, an operational athlete cannot be a one-trick pony. He or she needs to reach superior levels in several relevant fitness measures:

Aerobic conditioning: operational athletes need to be able to sustain moderate activity for extended periods of time. They are frequently tested in their ability to run, swim, or ruck over long distances against the clock.

Anaerobic work capacity/strength endurance: operational athletes need to be able to produce high outputs of intense work over very short periods of time, e.g., hauling heavy gear up several flights of stairs while still being able to perform their jobs afterwards.

Maximum Strength: operational athletes need to be strong enough to carry heavy loads (think of paratroopers rucking 100-pound packs) and/or produce overwhelming force (think of SWAT team members breaking down doors).

(C) SIMULTANEOUSLY

The operational athlete needs to be able to deploy these various fitness attributes all at once, within the same day or even within minutes. For example, a SWAT team member may need to be on his or her feet for hours during a stand-off situation and then be called upon to rush up several flights of stairs under a load of equipment in order to force entry and possibly go "hands on" with an assailant. Endurance, anaerobic capacity, and max strength are all called for in that same mission.

(D) AT ANY GIVEN TIME

The operational athlete doesn't have the luxury of a seasonal approach. He or she can't train like a powerlifter prepping for a meet, focusing exclusively on one attribute for sixteen weeks even to the detriment of all other attributes. When your job (and even your life) hinges on excelling across multiple fitness domains, you cannot approach training with an in-season vs. an off-season mentality. You must always be ready "to compete" at the top of your game in all aspects of fitness.

These four components show that the operational athlete faces a classic multi-variable problem. The operational athlete cannot afford a single-minded focus on any one fitness attribute. He or she needs to excel at all of them simultaneously. You can't go all-in for maximum strength and put on twenty pounds of body weight along the way when you need to run 1.5 miles in 9:00 for your next PFT. You can't push yourself beyond thirty pull-ups if that means you will be too weak to haul your gear. **The puzzle is finding a way to balance your efforts toward these different goals, not all of which necessarily work well together**. The simultaneous needs for max strength, aerobic endurance, and anaerobic work capacity are jealous mistresses that the operational athlete must placate.

Keep in mind that fitness is merely one part of an even larger puzzle for the operational athlete. He or she doesn't just need to pass physical standards but must also be good at the job. Skills practice, special courses, and working long and irregular hours all make additional demands. Factor in an attempt to have a personal life, and the operator is in risk of being torn to pieces by these competing demands. You might say that the operational athlete has many mouths to feed. So how do we perform this tenuous balancing act?

THE TACTICAL BARBELL SOLUTION

The primary puzzle for the operational athlete is to find a way to balance all of these demands, and *Tactical Barbell* and *Tactical Barbell II* provide a definitive solution to that riddle. These books are very detailed manuals, and I won't pretend to summarize them here. Studying them in detail might be the best thing you can do for your fitness progress, especially for those of you who are tactical professionals. Nevertheless, I want to distill a few key principles from *TB* and *TB2* that are particularly applicable for the ageless athlete.

THE LOWEST EFFECTIVE DOSE

First and foremost, the training plan for the operational athlete needs to run on a principle of extreme efficiency. He or she cannot afford to waste a single step. Any exercise, workout, or drill that doesn't advance the ball has no place in the operator's scheme. If you can get what you need out of three sets of squats, then any more is just draining your energy for your unit PT tomorrow morning. If you can maintain the endurance levels you need with a long run every two weeks, then anything more is a useless expenditure of resources you could put toward your lagging deadlift. If you don't need all those burn-out callisthenic finishers to get to your push-up numbers, then why be sore for tomorrow's skills training?

Read a lot of the typical fitness manuals on the market and you will get the impression the main idea is to find a way to pack as much training as you possibly can into a week. Tactical Barbell flips that mentality. The operational athlete asks herself how she can get by with less training. What is the *least* I can do and still excel in a particular domain? **Anything more than the least necessary is a needless drain on your progress in other areas.** If you read *TB* and *TB2*, you will occasionally find K. Black capturing this notion by referring to the **"lowest effective dose."**

Note well: Doing the **least necessary** is not the same as doing **very little**! The Lowest Effective Dose Principle is not an excuse to get you out of putting the work in. It's just the opposite. The idea is to put no more work into any one area than necessary so that you have enough left in your tank (in terms of both time and energy) to devote to progress in other domains. Training smart and efficiently is not the same thing as taking it easy. Moreover, the least necessary amount will vary depending on the kind of operational athlete. For example, an Army Ranger's least necessary is going to be a lot more than a fraud investigator's.

MULTI-PHASE PROGRAMMING

It is easier to address some variables simultaneously than it is others. For example, working on your maximum strength while addressing your anaerobic capacity works pretty well, and aerobic endurance and strength endurance are a match made in heaven. Attempting to make maximum strength progress while you are trying to get your 10K time up to par is not likely to end terribly well for most of us.

The problem is solved by multi-phase programming. The idea is to break up your annual training plan into phases emphasizing different attributes while maintaining others. Here's the way this works for the standard TB trainee:

- 8-12 weeks of **base building**, a phase emphasizing aerobic and strength endurance and maintaining maximum strength and anaerobic capacity.

- Indefinitely repeated 6-week blocks of a **continuation** protocol emphasizing max strength and anaerobic capacity while maintaining aerobic and strength endurance.

While you are building your endurance base (which is something just about everybody should do!), you put your maximum strength and anaerobic capacity in a holding pattern. You won't neglect these attributes. Strength and anaerobic capacity will get just enough attention necessary to keep all your hard-earned ground, but they aren't the main event in this phase. Once your endurance reserves are full, you go into a continuation protocol where strength and anaerobic capacity get the lion's share of attention. You give your endurance attributes some attention as needed depending on your goals/job requirements.

The multi-phase approach also has the advantage of allowing for specialization. Suppose you are a paratrooper who needs a lot more in the way of endurance attributes. Continuation can be tailored to suit those needs. Likewise, a SWAT team member's demands might stray more toward maximum strength. Continuation can be set up to take those priorities into account. Whatever way a particular operational athlete decides to play it to suit his or her needs, the base-continuation approach allows him or her to set certain variables as higher priorities without ruining everything else. By following a base-continuation cycle, all the attributes get what they need to progress without getting in each other's way.

STRENGTH WITHOUT USELESS HYPERTROPHY

When it comes to strength training, one of the common concerns for operational athletes is getting too big. Tactical professionals often have rigorous bodyweight standards to maintain. More importantly, tactical professionals need to be nimble, so there is no room for any excess baggage. Many people interested in this sort of programming are involved in mixed martial arts, which always carries the specter of making weight. In the popular imagination there is a strong association between training for maximum strength and the extremely bulky (and heavy!) bodybuilder look, which leads many tactical professionals to raise the "But I can't afford to get too big!" alarm when the subject of strength training comes up.

The fact is that this association is completely unwarranted. You can get strong, very strong, without adding dozens of pounds of puffed-up mass. All strength training and subsequent adaptation is going to involve some hypertrophy, i.e., muscle growth. That's not a bad thing; muscle is not our enemy. The task is to eliminate or minimize the gain of useless, overly bulky vanity muscle, while still getting strong and muscular to some degree.

Doing forced-rep-super-drop-sets with sequences of three or four exercises is not the way to go for the operational athlete. Neither are twenty-rep squats or multiple high repetition sets with moderate weights (10x10, etc.). You aren't going to the weight room "to feel the burn." Not only do those kinds of workouts leave you too sore to do much else, they are also perfect for adding the kind of muscle you don't want.

Rather, the key is doing multiple low repetition sets with relatively heavy weights and long rest periods. If you keep the reps low, the weights heavy, and the breaks long, you will get strong and minimize unwanted mass gains. If you peruse the three standard Tactical Barbell maximum strength templates (Operator, Zulu, and Fighter), you will see that they all require somewhere between 3-5 sets of 1-5 reps for each barbell exercise per session. Moreover, the weights are relatively heavy, moving from 70%-95% according to a weekly cycle. In no case is a set ever taken anywhere close to failure. It's really just classic block periodization stripped down to the absolutely Spartan necessities craved by the operational athlete.

In addition to manipulating your conditioning load and food consumption, one of the keys to keeping unwanted bulk at bay is K. Black's **Golden Rule**: **"Thou Shalt Rest a *Minimum* of Two Minutes Between Sets."** Notice that the Golden rule states a *minimum*. You might rest even longer: three, four, even five minutes between sets. For example, I have found that four minutes is the magic rest period for me when my squats get a little heavy. Complete or nearly complete recovery between sets is essential to minimizing unwanted hypertrophy while maximizing strength adaptation.

Manipulating these principles is what lets the operational athlete couple impressive levels of maximum strength while meeting his or her endurance demands and body weight requirements. This is the recipe for getting strong without getting too big.

ANCIENT WISDOM

The central concept of ancient Greek ethical thought is **moderation**. For example, Aristotle uses the notion of moderation to define the wise man as a person who performs actions "at the right times, with reference to the right objects, towards the right people, with the right motive, and in the right way" because "this is characteristic of virtue."[11] In other words, wisdom is the disposition to do more when that is called for and likewise to do less when that is appropriate. The wise person is moderate, avoiding both excess and deficiency. He restrains himself, even in good things, when doing so is the best way to achieve overall better ends. **This willingness to do less (when appropriate) is what allows the moderate person to achieve balance: by sometimes doing less, he or she can achieve more overall by excelling in all of life's domains.** For the Greeks, moderation is central to living the best sort of life because it allows us to balance our desires, interests, and goals. Living well cannot be reduced to just one good thing, so we need to be able to pursue many good things with moderation.

The Tactical Barbell system is an application of this ancient concept of moderation to solve the problem of achieving multi-domain fitness. The Lowest Effective Dose Principle, multi-phase training, and the Golden Rule (along with low rep, high frequency, high intensity periodization) are all recommendations for **moderation in training**. The trainee following these principles restrains herself in certain areas, in order to do more overall. Sometimes she will restrain herself by running only once each week, so she has reserves to handle more sets of deadlifts, which is currently more needful. Later she might put heavy lifting in a holding pattern for a couple months so that she can get her running up to par. These are all exercises in restraint in order to achieve balance, and in that balance the multi-domain fitness excellence lies. **The integral relationship between balance, moderation, and overall fitness** will be central to all subsequent discussions in this book.

CENTRAL TAKE-AWAYS FROM CHAPTER 3

- An **operational athlete** is an individual required to excel in multiple fitness domains simultaneously at any given time.

- Tactical Barbell addresses the operational athlete's **multiple variable puzzle** by prescribing:

- The **Lowest Effective Dose Principle** for maximal training efficiency;

- **Multi-phase programing;**

- Strength training protocols that **maximize strength adaptation and minimize useless hypertrophy.**

- Tactical Barbell achieves fitness **balance through moderation**.

CHAPTER 4:
THE AGELESS ATHLETE

CHALLENGES FOR THE AGELESS ATHLETE

With the detailed concept of the operational athlete in the back of our minds, we now turn to the broader category of the **ageless athlete** who may or may not also be a tactical professional. Basically, I have in mind someone who is training in his or her forties and beyond. Though we do not define ourselves or our goals by self-imposed limitations, we should consider the particular circumstances we are likely to face so we can specify programs that meet our real needs. What we can achieve may not be limited by our age, but what we have to do to reach those goals may need special measures. For those reasons I'll begin with a discussion of some of the hurdles the ageless athlete needs to surmount.

"I'M NOT AS GOOD AS I ONCE WAS, BUT I'M AS GOOD ONCE AS I EVER WAS."

We are pondering that saying from the great American "philosopher" Toby Keith because it brings out well what I take to be the central confusion most people have about training in middle age: **they diagnose the problem as diminished performance, when the real hurdle is a greater need for recovery**.

When I was playing college football in my early twenties, we kept a pretty grueling schedule. For a couple weeks during pre-season camp we had two or three practices every day. During the season most mornings we were in the weight room; we had full-contacts practices in the evening; and then we played grinding games on Saturday. Maybe you had Sunday off, but often that was an extra conditioning day (depending on how Saturday went). Most nights you had study hall until late in the evening, and of course there was plenty of wasting time in the dorms until the wee hours. In short, sleep was not a big part of the equation, and nobody was terribly meticulous about his diet. The most sophisticated recovery measure available was a bag of ice, if something was swelling. We did this day in and day out, and it didn't seem that tough. At that point I could go full-throttle almost every day of the week without much trouble. By the end of the season I was ready for a break, but after a week of rest I was always ready to jump right into off-season strength training.

I probably couldn't do that now. The daily grind would catch up with me in a hurry. I'm still able to perform as well (in many cases even better) on a given day, but an all-out performance is going to cost me something for a few days to come. When I deadlifted 600lbs a couple years back, that was an all-time best lift for me (both absolutely and relative to my bodyweight), but I was a bit of a mess for the week that followed.

I've found something similar when training BJJ. I can keep pace with fighters half my age, even some pro MMA guys, when rolling on the mat. Don't get me wrong: they submit me repeatedly. It's not even close in terms of skill. My point is that I don't get gassed out. I can hang in there for multiple matches with little rest. The difference is that those guys are probably coming back to the gym for a second training session that evening, and I am going to take the day off tomorrow.

In short, at this stage in life you can perform at very high levels, even superiorly, but it comes at a greater expense in terms of recovery. On any given day I'm as good or even better in every fitness measure as I have been at any point in my life, but I would have a very hard time making maximal efforts several days in a row. Whereas in your younger days you might have been able to absorb punishment almost daily, now you need more room to recover before you are back to 100% after you push the edge of the envelope.

This doesn't mean that you necessarily need to do less than you are doing now. In fact, you can probably do a lot more than you think. I mean "more" in two senses. On the one hand, you can probably perform across a broader range of fitness attributes. Like an operational athlete, you can (even in middle age) obtain advanced or superior levels of maximum strength, aerobic endurance, and anaerobic capacity. You can do more things. On the other hand, you can probably handle a much greater volume of training. You don't need to settle for truncated, two days per week training programs, nor do you need to limit yourself to brief sessions. You can handle more total training as a middle-aged athlete than the popular imagination expects.

The greater need for recovery doesn't necessarily mean you are going to need to radically limit what you do (either qualitatively or quantitatively). **You just need to have a sophisticated strategy to address your increased recovery needs**.

HIGH MILEAGE BODIES AND OVERUSE INJURIES

If you are training in your forties and beyond, there is a good chance your body has suffered more wear and tear than that of a younger trainee. This might be because you have been on the planet longer, or it might be because you have accumulated some nagging or overuse injuries from years from prior training. Your **training age** (how long and how intensely you have been in the fitness game) is probably more important to defining your limitations than your **calendar age** (how many years you have been on the planet).

This definitely resonates with my experience. As I mentioned earlier, I picked up some nasty stress fractures in my lower back when I was playing football, and that is something I need to be attentive to. I have also developed a tendency to strain my Achilles tendon when my running volume goes too far. (Working on pose running has helped, but this issue still arises occasionally.) I can't ignore these factors. That's not a self-imposed limitation but a painful fact my body brings to my attention whenever I go too far. I can still go out and match my old 5K and deadlift personal records (and hopefully beat them soon!), but I have to play those cards sparingly in order to work around some high mileage issues. Of course you need to follow the advice of your physician when it comes to injuries, and your accumulated injuries are among the factors you need to account for, but they need not end the game.

INCREASED NEED FOR CARDIOVASCULAR FITNESS

Now that you are in a more advanced stage in the Game of Life, you are probably a bit more health-conscious than you were back in your teens and twenties. Moreover, you probably have a more reasonable sense of human mortality now, and even more responsibilities and concerns that lead you to care more about your longevity (dependent children, a spouse, long-term professional goals, etc.). Thus, even if you are the most inveterate meathead powerlifter (that for me is a compliment!), I bet you are interested in "working on your cardio" more. I hear that all the time from people wanting to get back into training. Addressing this need can be particularly tricky when also taking into account the high-mileage or overuse problems we just discussed.

THE STRENGTH, HYPERTROPHY, AND WEIGHT CONTROL PARADOX

It is hard to find a health-conscious person over forty who is not at some level concerned with controlling his or her bodyweight. I'm no exception here. As a recovering fat person, I'd be lying if I said that I never worry about the scale. Even people who have been lean their entire lives report some difficulties keeping pounds off later in life.

At the same time, there is a good argument to be made that people past forty do well to build a little extra muscle. A few pounds of muscle can catalyze hormones and stimulate metabolism, both of which help with a variety of performance measures and aesthetics. Moreover, all sorts of health and quality of life markers have been shown to improve with increased strength and muscle.[12] Trying to address all of these variables can yield paradoxical results. While you are hoping to see the scale stay level or go down, you are at the same time training in ways that stimulate muscularity and strength.

It should be fairly obvious that the ageless athlete has to perform a balancing act very similar to that of the operational athlete. The ageless athlete has no ready excuses for not achieving a high level of fitness, yet he or she must be ever conscious of an increased need for recovery. Moreover, the ageless athlete needs to balance cardiovascular development, muscle gain/maintenance, and maximum strength development. Thus, **the ageless athlete needs to put together a multi-dimension fitness regime very similar to what is required by the operational athlete**.

Of course there are a lot of fitness programs that do so, and they tend to scale things heavily toward older trainees. You could probably address your health needs with a couple treadmill and moderate weight lifting sessions each week, so why go with a program primarily aimed at professionals in need of *superior* levels of fitness? If you'd even thought to ask that question, you probably would've quit reading this book a couple chapters ago. I don't know how to motivate excellence for people except to show them what it is and hope that its intrinsic value is enough to move them. So, if you want to know why someone might want to achieve and maintain multidimensional fitness superiority into middle age and beyond, have a look at the Ageless Athlete Profiles that appear at the end of each section of this book. Knowing those possibilities, why would you go in for programing that presupposes the very self-imposed limitations that are holding you back?

With the challenges facing the ageless athlete in place (increased recovery need, overuse and accumulated injuries, and the hypertrophy-weight control paradox), let's return to our basic tactical barbell principles ("the lowest effective dose," multiphase programming, and Golden Rule) to consider how they can be used to address those needs.

THE LOWEST EFFECTIVE DOSE AS THE KEY TO RECOVERY

The operational athlete needs the Lowest Effective Dose Principle in order to maximize the energy and time he or she can spend on each point of a broad spectrum of fitness and professional demands. Notice that the principle works in part by *optimizing recovery*. Suppose Smitty is in his continuation block. He caps his squat sets to the bare effective minimum to make sure he is recovered for a hill sprint session tomorrow. Likewise, Smitty limits his long distance running to just once every two weeks so he has enough left in his tank for his higher priority strength work. For the operational athlete, managing recovery reserves is decisive.

Certainly there is a need for days, even weeks, off for recovery purposes. We will discuss that at length later. Nevertheless, efficiency in training is the high road to optimized recovery. You will need fewer days off if you don't waste your recovery resources on any unnecessary steps in your program. Just like the operational athlete, the ageless athlete needs to plan for austerity. **Cut your training to the very bone, and in the long run you will end up doing more.**

MULTI-PHASE TRAINING TO RELIEVE OVERUSE AND NAGGING INJURIES

A typical operational athlete following the Tactical Barbell system will not touch a heavy barbell for the first five weeks of his or her aerobic and strength endurance base building block. Likewise, that same athlete might not do a single push-up or go on a long distance run for weeks on end during continuation. This will vary depending on specialization, but different modalities are cycled in and out as the top priorities throughout the year.

I know that sounds like dangerous heresy to you meatheads and endorphin-addicted ultrarunners out there. This approach, however, will make for better long-term progress, not the least reason for which is that it will cause you to spend less time healing those nagging overuse injuries. When the time for your annual base building block comes around, your body probably could do well to have a break from heavy weights and the sprints. Your shoulders, back, knees, or whatever ails you will recover and rebound after a break from loaded barbells and pounding on the track. Likewise, all the little ticks people aggravate or pick up from lots of long duration endurance work get plenty of time to heal during continuation.

I initially had a hard time trusting this concept. For me the problem was an addiction to long endurance sessions. Even when I wasn't in a base building phase, I was still forcing in at least two 60+ min runs, swims, or bike rides every week, on top of my Operator max strength work and an Apex session. K. Black constructively called me out on this during our email correspondence:

"Just curious, you seem to do a lot of LSS/E year round. I'm making assumptions based on our chats, so I could be way off here. But I gather that strength is a high priority of yours. Have you ever considered cutting down on the E/LSS or doing it as a smaller part of an annual plan instead of year round? Like 2-3 months of simple base building, and then switching over to a strength focused few months, with nothing but 2-3 HICS/week (or BJJ in place of a conditioning session). Basically abbreviated conditioning. You could really hit E hard for 2-3 months, run/swim 5-6 x week, simple max strength training on the side. Those benefits will stick with you when you transition to Black for the rest of the year, plus you'll get all the benefits of Black/HIC on top of that. The way I see it, anything beyond 3 months of frequent E for a civilian and you start getting into negative side effects territory. Keep one E per week or two in the rotation if desired. In my experience frequent year-round LSS/E impacts strength work. It can be done but it's an uphill slog."

Basically, I was doing too much endurance work alongside my strength and anaerobic workouts. I couldn't feed all those monsters simultaneously forever. I didn't feel any ill effects, and I managed to get away with this for a while. In the long run, nevertheless, it was going to hamper my progress or, even worse, cause burnout, hormone depletion, and injury. I knew all this, but I just wasn't pulling the trigger. I thought that as soon as I backed off the endurance work, I was immediately going to return to being a breathy powerlifter again.

After K. B.'s friendly intervention, I put my faith in the system and did a strictly Black continuation protocol (the *TB2* name for a continuation protocol emphasizing max strength/anaerobic capacity and minimizing/maintaining endurance work) for the winter/spring of 2016, followed by a summer base building period (culminating in a triathlon), and then back into Black for the fall and winter again.[13] As I write this in December of 2016, all my strength and conditioning numbers are equal to or better than they were a year ago, and, most importantly, I am having nothing in the way of problems with my nagging and overuse injuries. My muscularity and appearance are at their all-time best. Multi-phase programming should be part of your scheme!

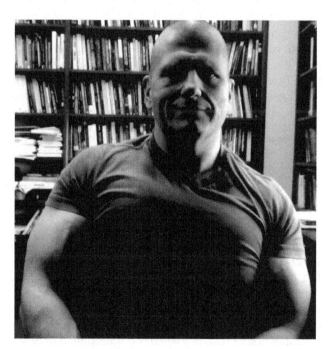

This is me (forty-three years old) the day I wrote this chapter, following several months of a strict observance of the standard Black protocol. Letting my endurance training take the back seat for a while didn't do me any harm!

THE GOLDEN RULE ALLEVIATES THE HYPERTROPHY-WEIGHT CONTROL PARADOX

We can stimulate a smidge of hypertrophy without going overboard simply by making small adjustments to the basic *Tactical Barbell* strength templates. For example, my preferred manipulation is to add a small amount of volume, i.e., either a couple extra sets or a rep or two to each set. During the Black continuation period I just mentioned, I added a few extra sets to each workout, especially on my upper body lifts. The results were fabulous. My strength numbers were up, my muscularity was the best ever, and my waist size was unchanged. I did gain just a few pounds, but it was clearly lean, and my condition and overall performance remained excellent. I got exactly what I wanted out of a small muscle gain. I will outline this program in detail in the next part of this book.

Note well: I left the Golden Rule untouched. Not once did I rest for less than two minutes during a max strength workout, and often I waited for as long as four minutes. I believe this is essential when adding volume for those of us who want just a smidge of extra hypertrophy. By keeping the rest breaks on the long side, you never go into the deep lactic acid release associated with typical mass gaining bodybuilding programs. Play a bit with sets and reps, but **the Golden Rule is inviolable**.

I hope the point is clear that training like an operational athlete, according to Tactical Barbell principles, is ideal for the ageless athlete. In making this case I have only given sketches and offered promissory notes on how to apply these principles to our specific case. That will be our task in Part 3, as we turn to programming for strength.

CENTRAL TAKE-AWAYS FROM CHAPTER 4

- The ageless athlete needs to accommodate a **greater recovery need**, work around **overuse/nagging injuries**, and make **small muscle gains with minimal weight gain**.

- Tactical Barbell principles offer ready tools to overcome these challenges:

- The **Lowest Effective Dose Principle** optimizes recovery;

- **Multi-phase programming** helps with overuse and injury recovery.

- Small changes in sets/rep while observing the **Golden Rule** make for reasonable muscle gains with minimal weight gain.

AGELESS ATHLETE PROFILE
MIDDLE-AGED MIXED MARTIAL ARTISTS

There is no better example of excellence across multiple fitness domains than mixed marital artists. To make it in the fight game you need superior levels of anaerobic work capacity, max strength, strength endurance, maximum strength, and an aerobic engine that doesn't quit, and all of that has to come together on an efficient physique that makes weight. Fitness is only part of winning in the ring. Fighters have to balance strength and conditioning with the demands of their skill work.

It's an achievement for an athlete to pull this off at any age, but there is an impressive cadre of middle-aged guys who compete at the highest level of MMA. Dan Henderson retired in 2016 at the age of 46, even though he was still competing as a top-level performer in the UFC. Daniel Cormier, in his late thirties, is (as of this writing) the reigning UFC Light Heavyweight champion. Anderson Silva, who has one of the most impressive MMA careers to speak of, is currently the number six contender for the UFC Middleweight title at forty-one years of age. Cormier, Henderson, and Silva are just a few examples of ageless athletes flourishing inside the octagon. These men aren't mere has-beens pathetically holding on to the old glory days. All three of these guys are or recently have been at the top of one of the most brutal and demanding sports there is.

Don't think it takes all the advantages and resources of a professional fighter with an entourage of trainers and coaches to cater to your every need. You don't get to enjoy that self-serving bias! I have a friend, Paul, with whom I train BJJ. He is 41 years old, a very busy restaurateur, an engaged father, and an absolute beast on the mat. He has had several professional MMA bouts, and he is preparing for another. His training schedule is rigorous, including a weekly swimming workout involving 50m freestyle sprints coupled with push-ups on the deck that makes my stomach churn just writing about it. Paul, at 41, is one of the most impressive physical specimens and overall athletes I have ever met personally, and there are guys and gals just like him getting it done in gyms and clubs all over the world.

PART 3:
STRENGTH PROGRAMMING FOR THE AGELESS ATHLETE

First, then, let us consider this, that it is the nature of such things to be destroyed by defect and excess, as we see in the case of strength and of health (for to gain light on things imperceptible we must use the evidence of sensible things); both excessive and defective exercise destroys the strength, and similarly drink or food which is above or below a certain amount destroys the health, while that which is proportionate both produces and increases and preserves it. So too is it, then, in the case of temperance and courage and the other virtues. For the man who flies from and fears everything and does not stand his ground against anything becomes a coward, and the man who fears nothing at all but goes to meet every danger becomes rash; and similarly the man who indulges in every pleasure and abstains from none becomes self-in-dulgent, while the man who shuns every pleasure, as boors do, becomes in a way insensible; temperance and courage, then, are destroyed by excess and defect, and preserved by the mean.

Aristotle, Nicomachean Ethics[14]

CHAPTER 5:
HOW STRONG DO YOU NEED TO BE?

The strength templates I am going to discuss allow for a lot of variation in the volume and intensity. If you follow any of these, then you will have some decisions to make about how hard you are going to push yourself on any given day. Do too little, and you will not meet your goals. Do too much, and you are on the path to burnout, injury, and woe. Thus, we begin our discussion of strength programming with some reflections on what exactly you want out of your strength training. Until you come to that conclusion, you cannot possibly decide how much is too much or too little for you.

BY ALL MEANS GET STRONG!

Mark Rippetoe certainly spoke wisely when he famously claimed that "Strong people are harder to kill than weak people, and more useful in general." The notion that brute strength is advantageous for contact sports such as football, wrestling, martial arts, etc. is certainly obvious. No one is surprised by the fact that getting brutally strong is important for physically controlling an opponent, and for some of these sports strength might even be a decisive attribute.

Rippetoe's point, however, has a much broader application beyond contact sports. For example, Lon Kilgore, Michael Hartman, and Justin Lascek make an interesting case that strength is a central factor for overall health and fitness.[15] They argue based on peer-reviewed literature that strength is actually an important foundational attribute for building muscular and cardiovascular endurance, so it is likewise an attribute that should be significantly developed by endurance athletes. The benefits of strength extend beyond the sports arena. Readers of tacticalbarbell.com hardly need to be reminded that many professions require a great deal of brute strength for both performance and safety, e.g., firefighting, law enforcement, construction, etc. Moreover, just being able to pick up something heavy without injury is an important practical ability for any self-sufficient adult. Kilgore, Hartman, and Lascek cite studies suggesting that "if you are in the top third of the population in terms of strength, you are less likely to die from all causes (disease, accident, etc....those in the lowest third of strength die faster than the other two thirds."[16] Of course correlation alone doesn't demonstrate causation, but it's interesting to see that being very strong is at least significantly associated with general health and longevity.

This shows that whether you are interested in sports, professional performance, day-to-day practical ability and safety, or even just basic health, it pays to get strong. Lifting barbells through compound movements is the most time-tested and effective way of building strength, so whatever your interests might be, the traditional barbell movements (squat, bench press, deadlift, and military press) should probably have a role in your training repertoire. Getting and keeping decent maxes in the traditional barbell lifts is a priority for any physical fitness regime, whatever your particular goals. This goes all the more for the ageless athlete who is attempting to extend high-level performance and vitality well into middle age and beyond. In short, whatever your fitness goals might be, you do well to spend some time under the bar!

DON'T CONFUSE NECESSARY WITH SUFFICIENT CONDITIONS

Logicians distinguish *necessary* from *sufficient* conditions. A necessary condition is something that must obtain in order for something else to be the case. For example, being an American citizen for at least 9 years is a necessary condition for eligibility to serve in the U.S. Senate. Thus, if somebody is not an American citizen, then he or she cannot be a member of the U.S. Senate. Notice, however, that being an American citizen for 9 years is not a sufficient condition for being a U.S. Senator. A candidate for the U.S. Senate must be at least 30 years old and a resident of the state he or she would represent in order to be eligible for a Senate seat, in addition to satisfying the citizenship requirement. Though 9 years of citizenship, being 30 years old, and state residency are together sufficient for Senate eligibility, they are each insufficient by themselves. To be eligible for the Senate, you must have the whole package. The point here is that something can be decisively important for a certain end (a necessary condition for that end), and yet not alone be enough to get you there.

Strength is a necessary condition for athletic performance, professional competence, everyday practicality, and maybe even health and longevity, but it is not sufficient. You probably are not going to be successful at reaching these goals unless you have crossed some threshold in strength development, but strength won't be enough all on its own to reach these goals. There is of course an exception to my claim: pure, brute strength (or some nearly associated attribute like power or explosiveness) is mostly sufficient for success in weightlifting, powerlifting, strongman competitions, and other narrowly strength-focused sports. In those sports, strength is not just one among a number of other attributes that are all necessary conditions, but by themselves insufficient conditions, for success. These sports are pure tests of strength.

Thus, unless you are training for a powerlifting meet (or some other pure strength competition), strength is just one among many attributes that are necessary conditions for reaching your goals. Strength is a necessary, though insufficient condition, even for the goals of a massive NFL defensive tackle. He definitely has to be brutally strong, but he also needs to be able to move, to be able to sustain performance through four quarters of grueling competition, and to master intricate physical skills. The NFL defensive tackle has to address many different needs in his training, not just strength.

Here is another example, taken from my own experience training BJJ. Frequently when I'm training jiu-jitsu I will get compliments from superior grapplers on my strength, **right after they submit me**! I always reply by pointing out that my strength might come in handy the next time I'm at a powerlifting meet, but here it's clearly not decisive! The point is that being strong might help me slow down these far more skilled athletes, but their better skills more than close the gap. Strength is necessary, but it is insufficient.

The vast majority of readers will fall into this category: strength is just one necessary condition among several others that are together sufficient for reaching your goals. Brute strength is an integral piece of your puzzle, but it is not all you need.

HOW MUCH IS TWENTY-FIVE POUNDS WORTH TO YOU?

You can't get too strong. After an MMA fight, finishing a marathon, going out on an emergency rescue call, getting a top score on a PFT, or surviving a car wreck, nobody has ever said "Things would have gone better, if I was just a bit weaker." *All things being equal*, get as strong as you can.

That being said, *all things aren't equal*. Ask yourself how much difference would 25 pounds on your squat max make for succeeding at the tasks I mentioned above? Would squatting 500 instead of 475 really make that much of a difference for your next MMA bout? I doubt that it would be decisive because either way you're pretty darn strong, and you're likely more than strong enough to do the work in the octagon. What if you didn't have the endurance to go the distance against a very fit opponent? That would be disastrous. Thus, if you went all-out to get your squat up to 500 at the expense of building a decent endurance base in preparation for a fight, you would be setting yourself up for grave failure. You're not preparing for a powerlifting meet, so don't train like a powerlifter who needs to squeeze every last ounce out of his barbell lifts at a great cost to his other athletic attributes.

Here's my point: since strength is a necessary but insufficient condition for your goals, you must balance it against the other necessary conditions you need to address. For whatever reason, many of us tend to get a tunnel vision when it comes to strength, which leads to an overemphasis on strength over all other athletic and fitness attributes. This probably has lot to do with the fact that everyone has been asked at a cookout "How much can you bench press?" Rarely, however, has your time in a conditioning drill or steadfastness in a LSS run brought you a whole lot of "street cred." We have all seen inexperienced trainees on internet forums lamenting the risks that will come to their bench press max if they start LSS running. Unless such a trainee is a powerlifter, he probably won't need every single ounce of that bench press max to meet his ends, so he might do well to balance it against developing a sound endurance base.

Let me use my own case again as an example. Right now it would be crazy for me to emphasize brute strength over jiu-jitsu skill training. I have more than enough strength to do well at grappling, but my skills are poor. It makes very good sense for me to add another night on the mat, even if it costs me a strength session. That's fine because I don't need to bench 400 or to knock-out a bunch of reps with "The Beast" on my pull-ups to improve on the mat, and I can still keep those lifts at a very good level. Moreover, when I first started rolling, I felt a dearth of strength endurance, which led me to emphasis that attribute over max strength for a few months. That only made sense, since jiu-jitsu was my priority. After I got my strength endurance levels up to where I wanted them, I was easily able to rebound my max strength. It's give and take.

Once you realize that strength is a necessary, but insufficient, condition for your particular goal, you then need to determine what level of strength will be enough to reach your end. Certainly there are going to be some absolute strength demands necessary for your goals. It is a very good idea to get clear on what those would be, and do your best to *exceed* them. By all means get as strong as you can, but don't become myopic. That is, once you reach the level necessary for your goals, make sure that continued progress with the barbell does not get in the way of other attributes necessary to your goals. If you need to slow down a bit on your strength progress in order to get your running up to snuff or to improve other skills, then that is simply what it takes to make progress toward your overall goal. What's better: a 10-pound improvement on your deadlift coupled with overall improvement across the fitness/skill spectrum, or 30 pounds on your deadlift without that complete overall picture? For most of you I suspect that former is the better scenario, whereas the latter might be disastrous. At the moment, I'd trade those twenty pounds of progress on the deadlift for more time rolling on the mat.

Now might be a good time to give some thought to both what movements (squat, bench, deadlift, military press, weighted pull-ups, power clean, etc.) have the best carryover to your goals (and if a movement doesn't serve that goal, get rid of it) and what sort of one-rep max benchmarks would demonstrate that you have ample strength for your task. You can make it an absolute priority to *exceed* those benchmarks, but you also should be willing to slow strength progress in order to meet and exceed basic benchmarks for other equally important attributes. We will discuss detailed considerations along these lines in the following chapters, but for now I just want you to raise the question.

DON'T FALL FOR BAD EITHER/OR THINKING.

Please don't fall into the very common *false* dichotomy that tells us that *either* you can get brutally strong *or* reach great levels of aerobic/anaerobic fitness, but *not both*. That simply isn't true, however much you hear it said on the web (usually from the mouth of someone selling highly specialized fitness implements or programs). Of course you probably won't win many national level powerlifting meets while keeping your 5K time under 20 minutes, nor will you likely clip out a lot half-marathons in 90 minutes while maintaining an 800 pound squat (though there are some pretty impressive outliers in these cases). I agree, but there is an oft-forgotten middle ground here: getting to very good, though not necessarily elite, levels across the spectrum. In other words, unless you are striving to become elite in just one aspect, the hard choice among the options—strength, conditioning, and skill development—simply doesn't arise. You can get to good levels, the thresholds you need to cross for your goals, in many different modes of fitness. You can get very strong and very fit overall simultaneously, with well-honed skills to match. It just takes a great deal of patience and openness to a "one step backward, two steps forward" cast of mind.

HOW MUCH CONDITIONING DO YOU NEED?

Much of what I have written in this chapter can be applied to your conditioning programming too, or really any other fitness attribute that can come at the expense of others. In fact, my own LSS overdose that I discussed in the last chapter is a case in point. I was running, swimming, and cycling far beyond what was necessary for my goals. In fact, retrospectively I can see that it was actually detrimental to some of those goals: maximum strength, and recovery for my jujitsu training. I had failed to ask myself "How much endurance do I really need?" If I'm not prepping for a marathon, an Ironman, or an elite military selection course, then I need to ask myself why I am trying as though I were. Taking your conditioning to a high level is great (I love it!), but make sure it isn't taking away from other priorities. Conditioning, like strength, is a necessary but insufficient condition for your overall goals. Accommodate your conditioning load to the extent that it is actually a necessary means to your goals. Once it occupies any greater space in programming, it is probably taking away more than it is giving. Remember that, like the operational athlete, the ageless athlete cannot afford to take many false steps.

You need to accustom yourself to this sort of thinking if you are going to implement the Lowest Effective Dose Principle into your programming. At times you will find it difficult to stick to this mentality, especially if you are a "hard charger." I know that I often have that problem. Some days you will do less than you could have. You will walk away knowing that you had a couple more miles to run in you, or you could've hammered out a couple more 90% triples on the bench press, and you will feel like you are wimping out. That feeling is misguided. It is a result of immature, short-termed thinking. You're wiser than that; you're an ageless athlete! Over the long haul (a lifetime!), you will do more (much more) by sometimes doing less today.

CENTRAL TAKE-AWAYS FROM CHAPTER 5

- **Whatever your fitness goals**, maximum strength is likely something you need to address.

- Nevertheless, maximum strength is **a necessary but insufficient condition** for achieving your goals.

- **Scale** your maximum strength program so that it actually suits your goals.

- **Conditioning** should likewise be scaled to fit your goals in tandem with maximum strength.

CHAPTER 6:
STRENGTH TEMPLATES FOR AGELESS ATHLETES

DOES THE AGELESS ATHLETE NEED
A SPECIAL STRENGTH TRAINING PROGRAM?

In a word, "no." I have seen many ageless athletes thriving on some very high volume, high intensity, and high frequency strength training programs. The Smolov squat cycle is an insanely difficult thirteen-week routine that pushes you to squat three to four days each week at very high volumes and intensities. It is the epitome of heavy, high-volume Eastern Bloc strength training. At its cruel peak the infamous Smolov "calls for an inhumanely high number of squats in the 81-90% intensity zone: 134 lifts or a whopping 44% of the total load. You are going to top off with three sets of four reps at 95% of your current—not projected—max."[17] It is an achievement for any athlete, whatever age, to complete this cycle, but it has been reported that an all-natural, masters (over 40) powerlifter took his squat from 560lbs to 665lbs in one cycle of the program.[18] You really can do more than you think!

I'm not recommending Smolov as an ideal program for the ageless athlete, however much part of me wants to dare you to try it. The guy I mention above is a world-class powerlifter preparing for a competition. He probably didn't do much more than squat, eat, and sleep for three months. He also probably had an extended off-season or deloading period after his competition. That's all well and good, but it's a far cry from the multidimensional, anytime/anyplace fitness I take as essential for the ageless athlete. You aren't going to get much running done the day after you endured 134 reps of >80% squats. I mention Smolov not as an ideal but as yet another reminder of how open the possibilities are throughout your lifetime.

That being said, we should have an "if it ain't broken, then don't fix it" attitude toward strength training programs. If right now you are thriving on a particular tried and true program, then don't be in a hurry to mess with a good thing. Needless to say, "program hopping" is a juvenile mistake. There is no sense in switching for variety's sake when you are currently making good progress. If you are training just for the workout experience, then move from program to program at random. If you are in this game for results, then stick with what you know works.

As an aside, I have found that I typically need to run two complete cycles of a program before I can assess whether it works for me. The first time through a cycle you tend not to understand the system completely; you are often having to learn new exercises; you make small mistakes with loading and timing; and it is generally difficult to make decisions about variable elements until you really know what you are getting into. The first cycle, for me at least, is often a bit of a botch. The second time around you usually have all the details squared away, so you can now get a better sense of whether the program works for you. I wait until I have really nailed a cycle or two down before I make any final judgment. At the very least, if you have paid for a program, you might at least try to get your money's worth before going back to doing your own thing.

WHAT ARE WE LOOKING FOR IN AN AGELESS STRENGTH PROGRAM?

Suppose that you now believe it is time for a change. Maybe your progress has stalled for a long period of time, and you have made all the tweaks you can to your current program without avail. Maybe you are completely burned out—not having a stale week or two, but completely sick and tired of Old Reliable. What should the ageless athlete look for in a program? This isn't anything different from what any operational athlete needs, but I note two closely related priorities:

- A strength program that coheres with the trainee's other fitness demands, i.e., conditioning

- A strength program that allows for ample recovery, while also forcing significant strength adaptation

The first priority is important because of the multidimensional emphasis of the training approach we are recommending. Strength isn't our only priority; conditioning is always going to be part of the picture. If you plan your annual training program around base building/continuation alternating phases (as I strongly recommend!), then the amount and mode of conditioning you do is going to vary depending on where you are in that process. During base building, aerobic conditioning takes center stage, and strength gets less love. During continuation (for most of you), strength, muscle, and anaerobic capacity will be front and center. In the rest of this part of the book we will operate under the assumption that we are programming for strength during your continuation phase. We will discuss my recommendations for strength programing during base building in the following part. So what we need is a strength program that allows us to give more or less equal attention to *high intensity conditioning* (HIC).

In order to accommodate this priority, our strength program is going to be limited by our conditioning program in the **intensity** of the weights lifted (literally how much weight goes on the barbell), the **frequency** of the lifting sessions, the **number of sets** performed, the **number of repetitions** performed, and/or **the number of exercises** performed.

Now consider the second priority. We need to recover, but we also need to push hard enough to get stronger. This would be easy if it weren't for the first priority. Otherwise you could lift as much and as hard as you want, and then then sit around for the rest of the week and recover. Think of our example of the master powerlifter following the Smolov program above. That won't work for us because we plan to be running hill sprints on our "off" days!

A very popular way of dealing with this problem is to cut down on the frequency of sessions and the number of sets performed, while still keeping the intensity fairly high and pushing hard for "rep maxes." On this sort of scheme the lifter will perform 2-4 sets at, say, 85% for 3 repetitions, and then push a final set at that same weight for as many repetitions as possible just short of failure. Maybe the lifter will get 8 reps on the final set, leaving one or even just a half rep in "the tank." The idea is to try to set an *estimated* 1-rep max personal best based on this final all-out set. This approach has been immensely successful, and I trained using such programs for years.

I do, nevertheless, recommend against this method for the ageless athlete for two reasons. First, I found that pushing for rep maxes on heavy lower body lifts was a recipe for burnout and injury. My squat and deadlift (especially the squat) made good progress using this method, but there were a lot of bumps in the road. Pushing for rep maxes on the squat and deadlift, especially when you start working with advanced or even elite weights, is going to become costly in the long run. You may get away with this in the short run, but down the stretch it will probably catch up with you. Rep maxes work better for beginning/intermediate lifters, but as you advance and the weights start getting heavy, it probably isn't a sustainable practice.

Second, I did not make very good progress on my bench press and my overhead press using the rep max method. I have found that these lifts just need greater frequency, and when you are pushing for rep maxes it is very difficult to provide that frequency. If I pushed for a rep max on a given lift on Tuesday, there was little chance I was going to be able to do much with that lift by Thursday. Since my frequency for any given lift went way down, it's not clear that there was any net gain of adaptation when compared to other programs that allowed for more frequent sessions without rep maxes.

For example, supposed I worked my bench press at 85% for three sets of 3 followed by a rep max of 8 reps. That yields 17 total reps on the bench press for that workout. That's not bad for a single workout, but that is probably the only bench press workout

I will be able to handle productively that week because of the all-out rep max set. Now suppose that I train the bench press for three sets of three reps at 85%. That's only 9 reps of volume in that workout, so we come out worse in terms of forcing adaptation within a single workout. Notice, however, since I only hit nine reps in that initial workout, I can now easily recover and come back for additional bench press sessions in the same week, probably as many as three total sessions using the same scheme. This approach yields 27 total reps at 85% for the week. That's a lot more opportunity for adaptation, which I have found leads to a lot better long-term progress. Thus, **by limiting the number of reps within a session, we actually come out ahead for our total reps for the week**. It's a real-world case of the proverbial "less is more." This is the sort of efficiency the Lowest Effective Dose Principle demands.

Keep in mind that you are likely to be much fresher the following day after a limited volume session than you will be after really pushing hard for a rep max. Thus, we should be suspicious of a rep max program when we consider our need to have a strength training approach that coheres with a serious conditioning protocol. Your mileage might vary, but I now stay away from rep maxes, except when I do an occasional test for progress. We will discuss my approach along those lines below.

Remember also that we don't want to go over the top in terms of hypertrophy. Generally speaking, you will see much bigger gains in muscle mass when working in the 8-12 rep range. Working in the 1-6 rep range will put much more emphasis on strength adaptation, while limiting, though not eliminating, hypertrophy. Moreover, sticking to smaller sets (1-6 repetitions) will cause less soreness and allow for easier recovery and a higher frequency of training.

OPERATOR AND ZULU FOR THE AGELESS ATHLETE

So what have we learned thus far? Our ideal is a **high frequency, high intensity** (heavy, 70-95%), but **relatively low rep/set** scheme. In the Tactical Barbell community, we typically realize this ideal in either the **Operator** or **Zulu** templates.[19] I am writing under the assumption that the reader is broadly familiar with the Tactical Barbell system, but some review might be helpful. Here is the basic scheme for Operator:[20]

OPERATOR TEMPLATE

DAY	WEEK 1	WEEK 2	WEEK 3	WEEK 4	WEEK 5	WEEK 6
1	3-5 x 5/ 70%	3-5 x 5/ 80%	3-4 x 3/ 90%	3-5 x 5/ 75%	3-5 x 3/ 85%	3-4 x 1-2/ 95%
2						
3	3-5 x 5/ 70%	3-5 x 5/ 80%	3-4 x 3/ 90%	3-5 x 5/ 75%	3-5 x 3/ 85%	3-4 x 1-2/ 95%
4						
5	3-5 x 5/ 70%	3-5 x 5/ 80%	3-4 x 3/ 90%	3-5 x 5/ 75%	3-5 x 3/ 85%	3-4 x 1-2/ 95%
6						
7						

In short, with Operator, you are going to lift barbells three sessions each week, separated by at least 48 hours. You cycle through 70-95% intensity (in two three-week waves), doing 3-5 sets of 1-5 reps. The trainee following Operator employs a cluster of 2-3 barbell exercises. This is high frequency, high intensity, low rep strength training at its brutally efficient best. Operator is the standard approach for operational athletes using the Tactical Barbell system, and it is likely the most popular template even among recreational trainees (like me!).

Here is the basic scheme for the intermediate/advanced version of Zulu:[21]

ZULU I/A

DAY	WEEK 1	WEEK 2	WEEK 3	WEEK 4	WEEK 5	WEEK 6
1	A 3-5 x 5 70%	A 3-5 x 5 80%	A 3-5 x 3 90%	A 3-5 x 5 75%	A 3-5 x 3 85%	A 3-5 x 1-2 95%
2	B 3-5 x 5 70%	B 3-5 x 5 80%	B 3-5 x 3 90%	B 3-5 x 5 75%	B 3-5 x 3 85%	B 3-5 x 1-2 95%
3						
4	A 3-5 x 5 70%	A 3-5 x 5 80%	A 3-5 x 3 90%	A 3-5 x 5 75%	A 3-5 x 3 85%	A 3-5 x 1-2 95%
5	B 3-5 x 5 70%	B 3-5 x 5 80%	B 3-5 x 3 90%	B 3-5 x 5 75%	B 3-5 x 3 85%	B 3-5 x 1-2 95%
6						
7						

Following Zulu, the trainee employs a "heavier" cluster (maybe as many as six exercises) broken into "A" and "B" workouts. Suppose our trainee organizes his or her program such that workout A is squat/bench press/weighted pull-ups; and workout B is overhead press/barbell row. He or she then performs the squat/bench press/weighted pull-ups on Day 1, and overhead press/barbell row on Day 2, etc. for the entire six-week cycle. The intensity and set/rep scheme waves similarly to what we saw above for Operator. The Zulu trainees gets to work with more lifts, and he or she gets a greater overall frequency of strength training, though there is some tradeoff because the frequency per lift goes down (from three days/week to two days/week) when compared with Operator. Even though with Zulu you dedicate more days to strength work, Zulu sessions (often with just 1-2 barbell lifts per day) leave a lot of time and energy for a subsequent conditioning workout or skill training on the same day.

Either of these templates is superb for the ageless athlete. You get everything you want with both options, i.e., high frequency, high intensity, low rep, periodized strength training that leaves plenty of room to accommodate your conditioning needs. I have used them both to good effect.

Nevertheless, I want to make a case for Operator over Zulu. Don't panic. There are a lot of Zulu devotees out there, and all the templates I recommend below will have Zulu options. I just want to explain what initially led me to move from Zulu to Operator.

I played around with the comparative arithmetic between Operator and Zulu I/A. When you look at the total volume for *a single lift* over the course of a six-week block (assuming you do the maximum allowed number of sets in every session), Operator comes in at 330 reps and Zulu I/A yields 230 reps. You get 100 more reps of total work for that lift per block. That's a lot more opportunity for adaptation to that exercise. Moreover, when you look at how the two templates compare for volume at various intensity levels, Operator comes out on top again. E.g., at 95% Operator gives you 24 reps/cycle while Zulu I/A gives you 20. Here's the point: when we focus on the total work for *a single lift*, in terms of both volume and intensity, Operator delivers more efficiently than Zulu I/A.

Now consider the two templates in terms of the total volume of repetitions for all lifts combined in a given cluster. If you assume that our Operator trainee is using a three-lift cluster, then he or she will total 990 repetitions per cycle (once again assuming he or she takes each workout to the max number of sets). On the other hand, with a four-lift cluster, the Zulu trainee will come in with 920 total repetitions. Operator continues to dominate. If we assume our Zulu trainee is using a five-lift cluster, Zulu I/A tops Operator with 1150 total repetitions. Of course Operator still delivers more repetitions per lift.

Thus, the bottom line is that Operator delivers a more efficient strength punch. The Operator trainee probably gets in more high quality strength work with **more time between sessions for recovery or work on other attributes**. This is exactly what we are looking for to help the ageless athlete flourish.

You might want to work on developing a greater range of lifts, e.g., you can't bear to let the overhead press go while giving your bench press attention. Maybe strength is very high on your list of priorities, and you want those extra 230 reps/block that Zulu I/A with a five-lift cluster can deliver, or you are a committed gym rat who simply likes putting more time in the weight room. In these scenarios, Zulu will probably be your thing.

I have found that using Zulu with four-lifts or an even more austere cluster can be very useful when life or other priorities are demanding. When my teaching schedule demands that I get my strength work taken care of quickly, I find it easy to get in the gym very early in the morning to knock out some squats/weighted pull-ups and get on with the day. At those times, Zulu is just what the doctor ordered. Likewise, when I am able to add extra BJJ training sessions to my week, but I don't want to take the plunge and go to Fighter (a twice weekly TB strength template), Zulu with a minimalist cluster is perfect. I can perform one or two lifts in the morning but still be very fresh to roll later in the day. Thus, Zulu definitely has its uses, but overall I recommend that you make Operator your default template, at least when you are starting out with this style of strength training.

OPERATOR I/A:
TWEAKING OPERATOR FOR THE AGELESS ATHLETE

K. Black has developed an intermediate/advance version of Operator with an eye to meeting some particular needs. First, as you progress and the weights get heavier, it can become a bit harder to keep up with the pace of standard Operator. A bit more maneuvering to recover between strength sessions can be quite helpful. More advanced trainees are better at making decisions about their volume and intensity. They know their bodies' capabilities well, so they can decide when to push and when to back off. Giving that kind of trainee some room for independent decision-making is a good idea. Moreover, a lot of operational athletes work floating schedules and long/odd hours that can make the rigors of the standard Operator schedule difficult to follow. K. Black's solution to these problems is to introduce variability into the Operator scheme both in terms of the set/rep/intensity plan and in the number of days between strength training sessions:[22]

Instead of the normal 48-hour spacing between Operator sessions, the trainee now adopts a floating schedule that allows for **up to** 72 hours between sessions. You have the variability to lift every other day or every third day.

Instead of limiting each session to five sets/lift, the trainee now has the option of working **up to** as many as ten sets per lift.

The intensity is based on a 75-80-85/90% three "week" wave. The trainee does five repetitions/set when working in the 75-80% range, and three repetitions/set when working in the 85-90% range. It is also up to the trainee to decide how many days (if any) to work with 90%.

In summary, the Operator I/A trainee works his or her way through three workouts at 75%, and then three workouts at 80%, and then three workouts at 85/90%. The workouts are spaced according to the trainee's schedule, recovery from the last lifting session, and other training demands. Push when you want/need to (in terms of volume, intensity, and/or frequency), and likewise back off when you deem it appropriate. Once you work your way through two 75-80-85/90 waves, either test or force progression. Operator I/A is highly intuitive, and most people who have worked with Operator for a long time probably make similar tweaks on their own.

Operator I/A is ideal for the ageless athlete, and this is how I usually structure my strength training for the continuation phase. Because you are "Not as good as you once were, but as good once as you ever were," you want to be able to push your performance when the spirit moves you, but you also want the latitude to take more time to recover from doing so. Since you are likely an advanced trainee (if not in terms of athletic development, then at least in terms of practical maturity), you will probably thrive on all the variability in decision-making. The slightly friendlier percentages will once again ease recovery.

Finally, with all the latitude to add volume in Operator I/A, you have a means for adding that touch of hypertrophy the ageless athlete needs, without going too far. I have found Operator I/A particularly helpful in that way. When I want to work on muscling up a tad, I just add a few extra sets to my strength sessions. You could also do six reps instead of five on 75% and 80% sets for a block or two. You will be surprised what a difference a small tweak like a couple extra sets or a few reps each workout can make. That's part of the magic of high frequency strength training: very small adjustments make for big results when projected over time. I have found extra volume on weighted pull-ups in the Operator I/A scheme is a particularly effective way to catalyze muscle growth in the upper body. Just remember that when you start adding sets or reps, the Golden Rule (**at least** two-minute rest periods) is still in place.

You don't need to take 72 hours of rest between your Operator I/A workouts. That's just a card you have up your sleeve. For the most part I still take 48 hours between Operator sessions (see my training log in Chapter 9 below). My BJJ classes and certain family and professional obligations are hung on definite days of the week, so there are days that I don't want to push longer max strength workouts onto. Thus, for me it works (as much as possible) to keep the three sessions/week schedule in place. When I feel beat up, sick, or if an emergency arises, I "flex" a day and make adjustments to get back on track next week. The variability for the intensity/reps/sets is, however, absolutely integral to my approach now.

The Bottom Line: for the ageless athlete, the ideal strength training template is Operator I/A.

CENTRAL TAKE-AWAYS FROM CHAPTER 6

- There is **no absolute need for a specialized program** for the ageless athlete.

- Whatever program you select, you should prioritize **high frequency, high intensity, lower rep schemes**.

- Schemes built around **rep maxes have a very limited shelf life** for ageless athletes.

- **Operator I/A is close to the ideal** for the ageless athlete.

CHAPTER 7:
CLUSTERS, ACCESSORIES, AND KETTLEBELLS

SELECTING YOUR CLUSTER:
FINDING HIGH YIELD/LOW RISK INVESTMENTS

There's a theme emerging that I'm sure you have noticed: efficiency is the cornerstone for a lifetime of productive training. We need to pick a cluster of main strength exercises that falls in line with this insight. I suspect that if you are reading this book, then you don't need a reminder that any serious strength training program needs to be built around big compound movements: squat, deadlift, bench press, overhead press, weighted pull-ups, barbell rows, weighted dips, etc. The question is which of the big lifts should be used to construct your cluster. These movements all have great benefits, and any one of them will be hard to let go for the confirmed gym rat.

Your first priority is covering all your bases. You minimally need a squatting motion, an upper body pressing motion, a hip hinge motion (think deadlift), and some sort of upper body pulling. This leads to some dicey decision-making when you set up your Operator cluster. You get at most three main lifts, and you need to cover four bases. If you are a Zulu devotee, then life is a bit easier. You can get away with four, five, or even six main movements in your cluster, so you won't have to make so many hard choices. Nevertheless, the more movements you stack into your cluster, the more you strain your recovery reserves and energy to devote to other attributes. Thus, even with Zulu you have good reason to economize as much as possible.

I think about this issue in much the same way you might think about a financial investment. Putting your money into an endeavor that is risky and doesn't yield much is irrational. Putting your money into something that is low risk and high yield is the ideal. We want to strive for the same sort of ideal investment when selecting lifts for a cluster. Here's an example. I've always responded very well to the squat, even when I was a kid. The movement comes easily for me; I recover well even from fairly high volume and high frequency squats; and it carries over well to other movements and attributes. My deadlift grows very well from the squat, and my muscularity seems to be at its best when I am squatting frequently and heavily. This video of my deadlifting 500lbs x 5 was taken just after I finished a long period of very frequent squatting and absolutely no deadlifting:

https://www.youtube.com/watch?v=vG4BPFYy7wY

That was the first day I had pulled a deadlift in over twelve weeks! As my squat surpasses 500lbs, I can almost guarantee that my deadlift will approach 600. Squat is almost all upside and nearly no downside for me. In other words, it fits the bill as a high yield, low risk investment. Suffice it to say, the squat belongs in my cluster, and that's not negotiable. For me, the squat is the ideal investment for my "strength portfolio."

The deadlift, on the other hand, is a different story. Pulling from the floor is just about my favorite thing to do (at least in the gym), and it's probably the lift I'm best at (I've pulled just over 300% of my body weight). Nevertheless, it usually costs me more than it returns. Most of my serious lifting injuries can be traced to the deadlift. Whenever I have fallen into the burnout/overtraining doldrums over the years I can probably trace the problem back to deadlifting too heavily and/or too frequently. Moreover, I can actually advance my deadlift without pulling very often. Thus, the deadlift is a pretty poor investment for me, however much I enjoy doing it. Anyway, now I pull from the floor sparingly. Usually 1-2 deadlifting sessions in each six-week block, pulling 1-2 triples at 80-85% is about enough to keep my deadlift in good order, as long as I am playing my other cards well. I treat the deadlift much like you might treat endurance work in a Standard Black conditioning template, i.e., I sprinkle it in every other week or as needed. Occasionally, I will put the deadlift in my weekly mix to make sure my "pulling tank" is full. Everything has its season.

Before everybody freaks out, I am not making a general claim about the deadlift. There are a lot of people who can pull heavy and often. Frequent (even weekly) deadlifting is something that has worked out badly for me, but other people have no such problems. I have also known some people who simply cannot handle a lot of squats. My point is not to make a specific recommendation here, but to point out that **you will have to find out which movements are high yield/low risk investments for you**. This is something that will have to be done by lots of trial and error, but keep an eye out for "good buys."

If pressed to make a general recommendation, I would go with K. Black's standard Operator cluster (back squat/bench press/weighted pull-up), with occasional deadlifting (once/week or once/every second week), and kettlebell swings as a frequent accessory. That combination gets all the bases covered (squat, press, pulling, and hip hinge), and it has worked superbly for me. The bench press allows you to handle a lot more weight than other pressing options, which get you more strength adaptation, and the same can be said about the back squat as opposed to other variations. I am relatively new to the weighted pull-up, but it has quickly become a staple for me. It carries over to my BJJ practice very well (grip, pulling, etc.), and I find that it really helps with physique and muscularity. I haven't done anything like curls in a long time, but my arms have definitely "blown up" since I started doing heavily weighted pull-ups. I will make my case for the kettlebell swing below.

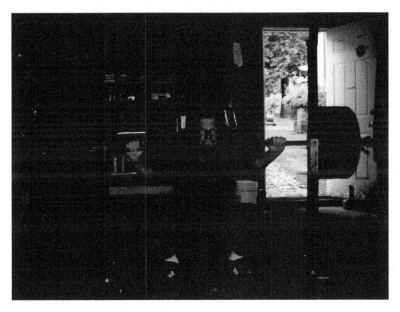

Here is Jim getting a good bang for his buck out of the squat.

As I mentioned already, when I deadlift less frequently, I play things intuitively by working up to a couple heavy-ish triples. For a much more systematic (and probably more effective approach) to the deadlift, see K. Black's "Incorporating Deadlifts" in *Tactical Barbell 3rd Edition*.[23]

VARIATIONS ON BARBELL LIFTS

I get a lot of questions about switching the traditional forms of the major barbell movements for variations—for example, swapping floor press for bench press. For the most part, my recommendation is to work with the full range of motion, i.e., traditional versions as much as possible. It is no accident that the squat, deadlift, bench press, and overhead press have become canonical elements of every tried and true strength training system.

There are two reasons that lifters move to variations. First, moving to a limited range of motion variation can overload certain muscle groups, which can help address a weak point. For example, someone stalling out just short of lock-out on the bench press might address that problem by focusing on limited range variations like the three-board press that overload the triceps at the top of the motion, and therefore produce a stronger lockout. Likewise, you will sometimes find a lifter who has a hard time breaking the deadlift off the floor doing his or her pulls standing on plates, in order to force a stronger initiation of the movement. These are all very effective techniques, but they also belong mostly in highly specialized programs designed for competitive powerlifters. The vast majority of non-specialists can get more than enough out of the plain old bench press without ever having to resort to doing four-board presses with 80lbs of additional chains. Maybe to break a frustrating plateau you might try some variations, but only as a last resort.

Second, you might need to employ a variation in order to work around an injury, a mobility problem, or an overuse issue. For example, I did a lot of analysis on my deadlift form a few years ago and found that at the initial positon I inevitably rounded my lower back. That's not good from a safety standpoint. (That may go a long way toward explaining my dysfunctional relationship with the deadlift.) I also found that limiting the range of motion by 1-2" made the problem disappear. Thus, I temporarily did my deadlifting with the plates slightly elevated, while I worked on correcting this problem in my setup. You might find floor press or narrow grip bench press to be effective ways of dealing with creaky shoulders. I will occasionally do a block using one of these variations as my upper-body pressing exercise. I also occasionally do a block of safety bar squats (to give my elbows and shoulders a bit of a break from the external rotation) or front squats (to give my back a break from some of the heavier squat loads). Here are some variations that might be helpful:

- Shoulder difficulties:

    Floor press

    Narrow grip bench press

    Pressing with a "football" bar

    Safety bar squat

    Overhead pressing with dumbbells or kettlebells

    Varied pull-up hand positions

- Back difficulties:

    Elevated deadlifts (shorter range of motion)

    Romanian deadlifts (done very strictly and carefully)

    Trap bar deadlifts

Front squats

Axle deadlifts

- Knee difficulties:

    Pushing/pulling a sled (to replace squatting)

    Front squat (to lower the load)

    High box squat (don't rebound on the bottom!)

    Trap bar deadlifts

I am not a big fan of trap bar deadlifts. Without being able to leverage the barbell against my legs, I feel very unstable at the top of the motion in a trap bar deadlift when the weights get heavy. I include it on this list because a lot of people have found it to be a lifesaver. Since your hands are positioned at your sides, you can pull from a much more upright position, which many people find to be a lot friendlier to the back. The motion ends up being something like a deadlift-squat hybrid, but it doesn't require terribly deep knee flexion. Thus, if you are having troubles with your knees, the trap bar might do some of same work as the squat for you.

The axle deadlift is an interesting option. My "axle" is just a 2" piece of pipe with makeshift collars welded on. Given the thickness and the fact that it doesn't rotate, this "barbell" is very awkward to pull. Even using an over-under grip, I can't pull nearly as much with the axle as I can with a standard Olympic barbell. The result is a very challenging exercise that greatly improves real world functional strength (GRIP!) but puts your back under a lighter load. At times when I've needed to give my back a bit of a break, I have employed this variation to good effect. As an aside, doing Pendlay Rows with an axle is a very challenging and effective exercise. Give it a try!

Whatever you might do with variations, I encourage you to **view them as corrective measures, and not ends in themselves**. The plan should be to use these variations as a means to eventually get back to the full range of motion versions. If you have mobility issues preventing you from doing full range of motion, then work to correct those problems. Of course, if you have injuries or long-term orthopedic troubles, then you might have to settle for a variation. The ideal, however, is to work with the **Big Four** whenever possible: Squat, Bench Press, Deadlift, and Overhead Press.

If your situation is such that you really have to settle for a variation long-term, don't panic. You can and will get strong using these variations. **What you have available and what you can safely do is the best option**, even when it falls short of the ideal.

ACCESSORY EXERCISES

I don't do a lot of accessory exercises. In fact, a lot of days my strength workouts are just squats, bench press, and weighted pull-ups—max efficiency. For the most part, I would prefer to **add volume to my main lifts rather than adding acces-sories**. Remember, we are striving to realize the ancient **ideal of moderation**. We only expend ourselves in what is necessary to meet our ends, and we prioritize only what is really important. Thus, you should first strive to get all you can out of the basic compound movements. Three more sets of weighted pull-ups are going to do far more good than all the curls in the world. If you have a lot of energy left over after that, then before dedicating resources to tricep pushdowns and cable curls, ask yourself whether you would be better to save that juice for tomorrow's trip to the track. The point is to moderate so that we can balance across fitness domains. If you are doing Tactical Barbell style conditioning (that typically includes calisthenics, kettlebells, core movements, etc.), then there isn't much need for any additional assis-tance work to smooth out muscle imbalances.

There are, nevertheless, three good "big bang for your buck" accessory exercises that I keep in my regular arsenal:

- Kettlebell swing

- Plank and Shank (standard plank followed by a static hold back extension)

- Dumbbell Farmer Carry

All three of these exercises emphasize the posterior chain, core, upper back, and (in the case of the swing and Farmer Carry) grip strength. Any holes in my normal cluster get filled in nicely with this package. As always, remember the Lowest Effective Dose Principle. Let's not overwhelm ourselves with a Farmer Carry beating on top of your regular lifting session. A little bit with all of these exercises goes a long way.

My suggested dose for the dumbbell Farmer Carry is two carries for about 100 yards round trip. Try to use a pair of dumbbells that puts you just shy of grip failure at the end of each trip. Once two 100-yard trips get easy, move to heavier dumbbells. If you prefer, you can go for time instead of distance (still stopping just short of grip failure). If you don't have the space, you can do static holds against the clock. Remember to observe the Golden Rule: take at least two minutes between sets.

The Plank and Shank is one of my absolute favorite nuggets from the Tactical Barbell Vault. It's the ultimate in a good exercise investment. You work a huge swath of muscles (posterior chain and the entire core) very safely and in an extremely time efficient manner. Holding the shank position will definitely test your will, so there is a mental toughness aspect to this exercise. Plank and Shank is an excellent bang for the buck! I like to do this exercise with some additional weight. You can use a weighted vest or backpack for the entire duration, or hold a weight for the shanking portion. If you have a partner, you can have him or her put some weights on your back during the plank portion. I generally use whatever weight I have in my vest for my weighted pull-ups that day. That saves a little time in the set up, and it varies the load. I tend to do just one all-out round of planking and shanking. I hold the plank as long as I can, and then I immediately go to the shank for max time. Trust me, if you really push a weighted Plank and Shank, one round will be plenty!

I'm going to go into detail on programming kettlebell swings in the next section, so I'll leave that issue aside for the moment.

Assuming that you are not using kettlebells prominently in your conditioning selections, here is how I suggest you work these accessories into your Operator scheme:

WEEK 1

Day 1: SQ/BP/WPU + KB Swings

Day 2: Conditioning

Day 3: SQ/BP/WPU + Dumbbell Farmer Carries

Day 4: Conditioning

Day 5: SQ/BP/WPU + KB Swings

Day 6: Conditioning

Day 7: Off

WEEK 2

Day 1: SQ/BP/WPU + KB Swings

Day 2: Conditioning

Day 3: SQ/BP/WPU + Plank and Shank

Day 4: Conditioning

Day 5: SQ/BP/WPU + KB Swings

Day 6: Conditioning

Day 7: Off

If you are adding deadlifts to the above scheme, I recommend that you do them only on Day 5 in place of the weighted pull-ups. You will need to gauge how much you can give to swings on Day 5, but you will likely be able to get some of them in.

If you are incorporating some serious swings into your conditioning (e.g., Apex, BOO, Meat-Eater 1, Meat-Eater 2, and Fobbit Intervals[24]), then I recommend the following approach:

WEEK 1

Day 1: SQ/BP/WPU + KB Swings

Day 2: Conditioning

Day 3: SQ/BP/WPU + Dumbbell Farmer Carries

Day 4: Conditioning

Day 5: SQ/BP/WPU

Day 6: Conditioning with KB Swings

Day 7: Off

WEEK 2

Day 1: SQ/BP/WPU + KB Swings

Day 2: Conditioning

Day 3: SQ/BP/WPU + Plank and Shank

Day 4: Conditioning

Day 5: SQ/BP/WPU

Day 6: Conditioning with KB Swings

Day 7: Off

For those of you adding deadlifts into this scheme, once again, put them only on Day 5. I haven't had any problems deadlifting the day before conditioning with swings. Your results may vary, so be prepared to make adjustments. You might need to adjust either the deadlift volume on Day 5, or the number of rounds/weight of the kettlebell swings on Day 6. Remember that with the swings, Plank and Shank, and Farmer Carries, you are getting a lot deadlift-type work. You can probably get by with just one set of deadlifts on Day 5 and make some progress. In fact, with this accessory package, you might find that you can get away with very infrequent deadlifting.

For those of you using an Operator I/A floating schedule, just alternate days with swings and days with Plank and Shank/Farmer Carries. When deadlifts come up, either drop or moderate the swing volume. If deadlift falls on a Plank and Shank/Farmer Carries day, either drop the accessories entirely or take them very easily.

For those of you working with Zulu, I assume you have deadlift in your heavy cluster, so I suggest something like the following:

WEEK 1

Day 1: SQ/BP/WPU + Swings

Day 2: OHP/Row + Dumbbell Farmer Carry

Day 3 Conditioning

Day 4: SQ/BP/WPU

Day 5: OHP/DL + Swings

Day 6: Conditioning

Day 7: Off

WEEK 2

Day 1: SQ/BP/WPU + Swings

Day 2: OHP/Row + Plank and Shank

Day 3 Conditioning

Day 4: SQ/BP/WPU

Day 5: OHP/DL + Swings

Day 6: Conditioning

Day 7: Off

Here too you will need to balance the deadlift and swing volume on Day 5. You might find that doing swings and Plank and Shank on consecutive days (1 and 2 in Week 2) is too much for your hamstrings. In that case, just do your entire block as Farmer Carries on Day 2, and add some extra core work as you feel you need it. If you are a deadlifting x 2/week person, then be attentive to whether you need to moderate your accessories on Day 2 and Day 5, as you are getting a lot of work for the posterior chain. There will always be some give and take.

INCORPORATING KETTLEBELL SWINGS

As you read in the first chapter, kettlebells were integral to my move toward multi-dimensional fitness. I have worked extensively with a number of kettlebell exercises: swings, snatches, C&P, Turkish get-ups, doubles variations, etc. Nevertheless, the basic kettlebell swing is the mainstay for me. The swing has been the one constant in my training program since 2006. Before you worry about incorporating more advanced kettlebell exercises into your package, ask yourself whether you really have milked the swing for everything it has to offer. I doubt that you can answer that question affirmatively. I have advanced to the point that I can swing the Beast one-handed casually, and I still don't feel the need to add much else to my kettlebell arsenal:

https://www.youtube.com/watch?v=pKF3GljL2lQ

One of the most frequent questions that I get on the Tactical Barbell forum is how to incorporate kettlebell swings into Operator. There are a lot of specialized kettlebell programs available, so if you want to go down that rabbit hole (and I'm not saying that is a bad place to be!), I suggest that you seek one of them out.[25] There are far worse ways to spend your time. I'm not going to go into anything quite so detailed. What follow are two very basic kettlebell swing programs that I have used in conjunction with Operator with good effect. I'm assuming that anybody looking for concrete programing for swings has them pretty high on his or her priority list, so both templates don't include deadlifts in the Operator cluster.

BASIC SWINGS PERIODIZATION

Suppose you aren't looking for a total kettlebell domination or even a novel challenge. For you the swing is just one more exercise in your cluster. If that's the case, let's not overcomplicate things. You are already working through a periodized scheme for your barbell exercises, so let's just apply that to your swings. This is simplest way to incorporate kettlebells into your template in a structured way.

Start with a kettlebell you are reasonably certain you can swing for 100 reps in sets of either 10L-10R one-handed (1H) swings or 20 two-handed (2H) swings **following the Golden Rule (at least two minutes of rest between sets)**. My preference is that you work with one-handed swings as much as possible on your strength days, and 2H swings on your conditioning days. In the former case, you will have the luxury to take as much time as you want to rest between sets, so you won't be in as much of a fatigued state. Therefore, you will be far less prone to dangerous technical errors that can arise with the less stable one-hand swing. That is a good time to help yourself to the benefits of the one-handed swing while mitigating the risks. When you swing in the midst of a high intensity conditioning drill, you will be fatigued and more error prone. In that case you will want the much more stable platform of the two-handed swing. All swings are good, so if you prefer the two-handed swings even on strength days, then go for it.

You may then follow this basic periodized scheme:

WEEK 1

Day 1: SQ/BP/WPU + 70 total swings (10L-10R x 3, 5L-5Rx1 or 2H/20x3, 10x1)

Day 3: SQ/BP/WPU + Farmer Carry

Day 5: SQ/BP/WPU + 70 total swings (10L-10R x 3, 5L-5Rx1 or 2H/20x3, 10x1)

WEEK 2

Day 1: SQ/BP/WPU + 80 total swings (10L-10R x 4, 5L-5Rx1 or 2H/20x4)

Day 3: SQ/BP/WPU + Plank and Shank

Day 5: SQ/BP/WPU + 80 total swings (10L-10R x 3, 5L-5Rx1 or 2H/20x3, 10x1)

WEEK 3

Day 1: SQ/BP/WPU + 90 total swings (10L-10R x 4, 5L-5Rx1 or 2H/20x4, 10x1)

Day 3: SQ/BP/WPU + Farmer Carry

Day 5: SQ/BP/WPU + 90 total swings (10L-10R x 4, 5L-5Rx1 or 2H/20x4, 10x1)

Your swing volume tracks the intensity of your week in Operator. This method is very similar to the way bodyweight exercises are programmed in *Tactical Barbell*: use a percentage of your max repetitions more or less parallel to the percentage of 1RM being used for that week in the strength template. Don't worry about adding the extra five percent swings during the 75-85-95 weeks for your barbell lifts. There is no need to complicate things, so we'll just round down to play it safe. The same goes if you are using Operator I/A percentages: go with 70-80-90. Life is too short to worry about five swings either way.

If you are using Zulu, the scheme looks like this:

WEEK 1

Day 1: SQ/BP/WPU + 70 total swings (10L-10R x 3, 5L-5Rx1 or 2H/20x3, 10x1)

Day 2: OHP/Row + Dumbbell Farmer Carry

Day 4: SQ/BP/WPU

Day 5: OHP/DL + 70 total swings (10L-10R x 3, 5L-5Rx1 or 2H/20x3, 10x1)

WEEK 2

Day 1: SQ/BP/WPU + 80 total swings (10L-10R x 4, 5L-5Rx1 or 2H/20x4)

Day 2: OHP/Row + Plank and Shank

Day 4: SQ/BP/WPU

Day 5: OHP/DL + 80 total swings (10L-10R x 4, 5L-5Rx1 or 2H/20x4)

WEEK 3

Day 1: SQ/BP/WPU + 90 total swings (10L-10R x 4, 5L-5Rx1 or 2H/20x4, 10x1)

Day 2: OHP/Row + Dumbbell Farmer Carry

Day 4: SQ/BP/WPU

Day 5: OHP/DL + 90 total swings (10L-10R x 4, 5L-5Rx1 or 2H/20x4, 10x1)

During Week 2, you will need to judge how your back/hamstrings feel when deciding whether you are going to do the Plank and Shank on Day 2 twenty-four hours after doing high volume, heavy swings. If need be, drop the accessories entirely on Day 2 or go with the Farmer Carry for the whole block.

Remember that you are following the Golden Rule for your sets of swings. The point of these swings is not conditioning but strength. Take your time in between sets. Recover as close to fully as your schedule allows. Aim for absolute technical perfection on every swing.

Keep an eye on your recovery during the 90 swings weeks because you will be squatting (and maybe deadlifting) pretty heavily those weeks, too. If you find that this is too much of a load, consider cutting down to just one day of swings that week, or just do 80% swings that week.

As we discussed above, if you are going to do a HIC that involves kettlebells (Apex, BOO, Fobbit Intervals, Meat-Eater 1 and 2, etc.), put that workout on Day 6, and skip the swings on Day 5. You will get more than enough swinging volume between Day 1 and your HIC.

Finally, if you are deadlifting, I recommend that you keep it to once each week when doing this kettlebell swing program. Either drop your swings the day you deadlift (if you are deadlifting, you probably don't need a second day of swings anyway), or cut the volume in half on the second day of swings.

THE 100 SWING CHALLENGE

If you want a little more in the way of excitement out of your kettlebell swing programming, here is something you can play with a bit. Pick a moderately heavy kettlebell for you, and set a goal to get 100 swings with that bell continuously— without putting it down. I've taken this challenge for a couple kettlebells, and here is how I have done it (in the following chapter you can follow how I used this process to get to swinging a 40KG KB, "The Bulldog," for one hundred continuous reps).

On the first day of the cycle, begin by swinging the kettlebell for as many reps as you can, pushing yourself hard without completely falling apart technically. Let's say you are using a 32KG kettlebell, and you get 45 swings. Take a good break (you will need it!), and when you feel sufficiently recovered, do the same thing. Let's suppose you get 30 swings this time. Repeat the process until you get to 100 total for the day. Let's suppose you do a set of 15 and a set of 10 to round things out. You will probably be huff'n and puff'n a bit from this series, especially if you push that first set. Thus, you will take it pretty easy on the second day of swings, do Plank and Shank or dumbbell Farmer Carries, or just include some swings in your conditioning on Day 6 (though you might want to use a lighter KB that day).

Here's how this will look in Operator:

WEEK 1

Day 1: SQ/BP/WPU + Swing – 32KG/45-30-15-10

Day 3: SQ/BP/WPU + Farmer Carry

Day 5: SQ/BP/WPU + Swings – 32 KG/10L-10R x 2-3

WEEK 2

Day 1: SQ/BP/WPU + Swing – 32KG/45-30-15-10

Day 3: SQ/BP/WPU

Day 5: SQ/BP/WPU + P&S or Farmer Carry

WEEK 3

Day 1: SQ/BP/WPU + Swing – 32KG/45-30-15-10

Day 3: SQ/BP/WPU

Day 5: SQ/BP/WPU

Day 6: Apex Hill Sprints (or some other kettlebell-based HIC)

Working toward 100 reps with a heavy kettlebell is taxing, so here we cut down on the frequency of your swing sessions a bit as you get to your heavier weeks for your other lifts. You swing twice in week one, only once in week two, and once with a kettlebell conditioning session in week three. On Day 1 of each week you will try to combine some of the sets from last week's Day 1. Probably you will combine the last two sets to get this: 32KG/45-30-25. If that's too much, don't worry. Just hang with what you did last week—patience. Sometimes you will find that the first set is really easy, so you can jump to something like this: 32KG/60-20-20. Great! Just don't rush things needlessly. Keep combining sets and/or increasing the initial set until you end up swinging your kettlebell for 100 continuous reps. The day you do that will be pretty taxing (your glutes and hamstrings might be a mess), so be prepared to make adjustments to your conditioning load that week. This challenge certainly makes a significant conditioning contribution.

Here is how the 100 Swing Challenge translates to Zulu:

WEEK 1

Day 1: SQ/BP/WPU + Swing – 32KG/45-30-15-10

Day 2: OHP/Row + Dumbbell Farmer Carry

Day 4: SQ/BP/WPU

Day 5: OHP/DL + Swing – 32KG/45-30-15-10

WEEK 2

Day 1: SQ/BP/WPU + Swing – 32KG/45-30-15-10

Day 2: OHP/Row + Plank and Shank

Day 4: SQ/BP/WPU

Day 5: OHP/DL

WEEK 3

Day 1: SQ/BP/WPU + Swing – 32KG/45-30-15-10

Day 2: OHP/Row + Plank and Shank

Day 4: SQ/BP/WPU

Day 5: OHP/DL

Day 6: Apex Hill Sprints

Remember that "32KB/45-30-15-10" is a just a hypothetical example. On Day 1, start with your best continuous set of swings (with good form), and then fill in with additional sets until you get to 100. As you can, combine sets and/or increase your initial set until you can swing your kettlebell one hundred times continuously.

- Practice wise investment strategy when selecting exercises for your cluster: **low risk and high yield**.

- When used **sparingly, variations of the tradition barbells exercises can be effective tools** for the ageless athlete.

- Limit accessory lifts as much as possible for ageless athletes, though there is a lot of value for the **Plank and Shank, Dumbbell Farmer's Carry, and the KB Swing** when using the standard Operator cluster.

- Consider programming the kettlebell swing alongside Operator using either **Basic Swing Periodization** or the **100 Swing Challenge scheme.**

CHAPTER 8:
PROGRAMMING RECOVERY

PREEMPTIVE ACTION

We all love to train. Frequently it's the most fun part of the day. On days I don't train, I find myself a bit fidgety. I don't sit still well; I'm distracted; and, frankly, I'm a bit irritable. I'd be lying if I denied that a big part of my self-esteem is wrapped up in my training, and I suspect that a lot of you would say the same. I definitely feel the absence of my workouts on my off days.

For these reasons it is hard to commit to off days. I understand that. I find it hard, too. Every fitness authority will tell you the value of recovery, but when you talk to them frankly, they will likely tell you that they, too, have learned this lesson the hard way. Remember, however, that moderation is the ideal we are striving for in constructing a fitness program. That means we need to restrain ourselves when doing that is what best serves our ends. This issue is all the more crucial now that you "aren't as good as you once were …." Recovery is our primary variable to account for. When you are younger, you have a lot more latitude for planning your recovery days. I tended to have a "rest as needed" approach. I would back off, maybe even taking weeks off from heavy lifting, but only when I really felt as though I were starting to hit bottom.

Now my recovery game needs to be a bit more precise. First, the "rest as needed" plan wasn't all that effective even back in the good old days. I suffered lots of problems with burnout, stagnation, and injury. Not surprisingly, my youthful powers of judgment weren't all that reliable. "As needed" usually happened after I had crossed the threshold of burnout, not before. Now that I'm older, I can't afford those sorts of errors as readily. **I can't wait for a problem to arise; I need to be proactive in making sure I get enough rest and recovery time**.

This requires an important mentality shift. Most of you reading this book are probably very ambitious, high achieving, competitive individuals who push themselves hard in all of life's arenas. In our more foolish moments, people like us think of recovery days as "wimping out" or "being soft." At the very least you probably feel as though taking time to recover is a concession or a necessary evil. At the root of this attitude is the sense that taking time off is something you have to accept passively, a necessary evil you suffer, or a lost opportunity.

We need to rethink that attitude. **Taking time to recuperate is not passive. It's an active way of taking charge of your long term progress**. By pushing the edge indefinitely and waiting for a problem to arise before you take preventative measures, **you are actually leaving your progress up to chance**. You are simply rolling the dice and hoping for the best. That's passive. **By planning and programming your rest time, you are taking control**. You aren't tempting fate; rather, you're asserting yourself as the governor of your training.

For a hard-charging trainee, planning and sticking to a program of scheduled rest can actually be the most difficult test of your personal discipline. I know that is true for me. My number one vice is doing too much, both within my workouts (more on that issue in subsequent chapters) and in my overall scheme. It is the truly seasoned and disciplined trainee who is willing to let up when it is appropriate, which is probably more often than you care to admit. That's not selling yourself short or "wimping out" but doing what it takes to make sure you will be good to go for decades. It's moderation!

Aristotle famously defined the virtue of courage as **the mean between the vice of cowardice and the vice of irascibility**. That is, the courageous person is someone who neither always runs away nor always stays to fight. He or she is wise in dealing with both fear and honor, and fights or runs when it is appropriate. Certainly courage requires us to stand and fight when doing so will actually do our cause some good. Likewise, courage also requires us to run away when doing so is what is best for our cause. Does this sound familiar? It is the application of the ideal of moderation to our dealings with fear and honor.[26]

What I am recommending here is the application of the Aristotelian virtue of courage to your training. By all means stand and fight when doing so is actually good for you. Be disciplined and get your workouts done. At the same time, there are days or even weeks when backing off is the appropriate action. Taking a day off isn't necessarily cowardice but can actually be the courageous action when it furthers you toward your goals more so than trudging on with an ill-conceived workout.

Think of planned recovery days or weeks as **preemptive actions**. You are striking first—before burnout, injury, or stagnation can have their way with you. You are taking the appropriate actions to reach your goals, and among those are actually measures to refrain from training. That's not wimping out; it's wise. It is wisdom that we should expect from an ageless athlete.

HOW MANY RECOVERY DAYS EACH WEEK?

You need at least one recovery day that is written in stone and non-negotiable. You need the guarantee that you will have a least one day to buffer against doing too much. I'm not saying you need to be a sedentary slob that day. Light recreational activity, yardwork, playing with your kids, and easy mobility work are fine. Just no weights, sprints, extended LSS, or anything of the like. Take a day off from your training completely.

Incidentally, I like to schedule my mandatory day off on a weekday whenever possible. My weekdays are busier professionally and often are for my family too. Thus, if I can hang a day off on a weekday, that gives me a chance to catch up on other tasks. On the weekends, especially if I'm willing to get up a little earlier, I have more hours I can put toward training and a generally more flexible schedule, so it makes sense to use those days for training. This doesn't mean you have to abandon your family on the weekends, if you get creative. It's not out of the ordinary to see me doing a fun run in a weighted vest between games at the youth soccer complex, and we regularly take the entire family to the track for Sunday Run Day.

I also recommend that you have a **variable rest day each week**. This gives you the latitude to make decisions based on how things are going that week. Of course, if you are running Operator I/A with the floating rest day, you have all the flexibility you need. It generally works best for me to keep my max strength days during the week on definite days, so I regulate my strength work by playing with the volume within the sessions. Where I build flexibility into my schedule is with my conditioning. Since I train BJJ too, here is my rule of thumb:

> 1-2 conditioning workouts (HIC or LSS) and 1-2 BJJ practices, **not to exceed three total sessions**.

Yes, I count BJJ as conditioning. Is it HIC? LSS? General conditioning? I don't know; the duration and intensity really varies from one session to another. I just chalk it up as generic conditioning. Notice that this rule of thumb doesn't mandate three total conditioning sessions. I won't exceed three sessions in any given week, but I don't require myself to do three conditionings. That is where the variable rest day comes into play. If I have a tough roll or go crazy with the squats, I will drop one of the HIC/LSS workouts that week. Likewise, if I miss a BJJ practice, I can either take another day of rest or fill in with an extra HIC/LSS. If I want to push really hard on conditioning, then I might need to limit my BJJ training that week or cap my lifting sets at the minimums.

If you don't have a practice like BJJ or some such to work around, **your rule of thumb should probably be 1-3 HIC/LSS**. Don't be afraid of doing even just one conditioning session when you need to. If you do go with three tough HIC sessions in a week, be prepared to restrain yourself in the weight room.

WEEKS OFF: THE 3-1-3-1 APPROACH

Typical Tactical Barbell athletes (during continuation) take a back-off week after a six-week or twelve-week block of training. That is a generally sound approach, but I have recently had very good results with more frequent back-off weeks. Right now, I take a **recovery week** every fourth week, so my schedule looks like this:

3-1-3-1

Week 1: Black+Operator/Zulu

Week 2: Black+Operator/Zulu

Week 3: Black+Operator/Zulu

Week 4: Recovery Week

Week 5: Black+Operator/Zulu

Week 6: Black+Operator/Zulu

Week 7: Black+Operator/Zulu

Week 8: Recovery Week

Notice that it now takes eight weeks to complete what was normally a six-week Operator/Zulu block. That's not a worry because we are in no hurry on the journey to lifelong excellence. Slowing things down in the short term is what will keep us in the game for the long haul. Knowing that I have a planned recovery week always on the near horizon lets me push a bit harder without worry. Don't do anything crazy, but you can get away with a few extra sets of weighted pull-ups or a couple more trips up your toughest hill when you know next week you won't have to do this again. I have found that the 3-1-3-1 approach makes a noticeable difference for the total volume of training I can handle (both strength and conditioning).

Notice that I have not called the "1" weeks "off weeks" but "recovery weeks." **I do stay entirely away from barbells and HIC during recovery weeks**. That is the key to recharging the CNS, joints, hormones, etc. I don't, however, always take those weeks completely off. I still go to BJJ practice, and either I roll an additional day or I work on some attributes I don't normally hit in my training, e.g., strength endurance or general conditioning. Easy week is also a good time to check in with a LSS session too. I recommend that you keep it to **no more than two workouts that week**, plus any other activities you might have (BJJ in my case), and remember **to keep the workouts easy**. If you have a flexibility or mobility protocol you like to follow (not a bad idea), incorporate that as much as you like. Here's what a recovery week typically looks like for me:

Sunday: Progressive Grip Circuit + mobility work

Monday: Off

Tuesday: BJJ practice

Wednesday: Off

Thursday: Quarterdeck Core + mobility work

Friday: Off

Saturday: BJJ practice

Or

Sunday: Brig Rat (1-2 rounds) + mobility work

Monday: Off

Tuesday: BJJ practice

Wednesday: Off

Thursday: Off

Friday: 30-60 min LSS swing + mobility work

Saturday: Off

So the rule of thumb for a recovery week is **no more than two general conditioning, grip, core, or LSS sessions**. Keep the pace chill and the intensity minimal/moderate. It is supposed to be easy without being stagnant. Do all the restorative, pre/rehab, or mobility work you like. Every other block, I recommend taking the second "1" week entirely free from any kind of serious training.

RECOVERY ROUTINE

Effective recovery is not merely a matter of taking the time to let your body's recuperative powers operate. You also need to take actions to help your body maintain those capacities. I don't have a terribly sophisticated recovery regime, but I have found that just a few consistent practices over the years have made a big difference for me. These practices are **sleep, diet, supplementation**, and **mobility work**.

Sleep. Getting at least 7-8 hours of quality sleep has proven to be all-important for me. When I skimp on sleep, I find that I just don't turn it around very well between workouts. When I was in graduate school, I could be "good to go" on a very truncated sleep schedule, but those days are definitely over for me. I have found that when I am disciplined in this manner, I can handle much more exercise; I need to take fewer days off; and I perform much better. I also find that when I am getting a very regular 7-8 hours of sleep every night I get fewer "junk food" cravings, and I find it generally easier to stick to my dietary plan. Higher frequency and higher quality workouts, and better dietary dispositions: it shouldn't take more than that for you to make sleep a big priority. I'm sure that the value of good sleep for recovery and athletic performance isn't new to anybody.[27]

Of course, when my kids were younger, this was all much more easily said than done. There are going to be times in your life when your family and job will make it very difficult, if not impossible, to get eight hours of sleep each night, or really any sort of regular sleep schedule. Now, however, for me my sleep habits are a question of priority, not necessity. That is, whether I get my eight hours each night is usually a matter of putting my sleep needs above other activities. I have to ask myself whether staying up to watch a movie or having an off-topic conversation at work when I should be grading a stack of papers (thereby insuring that I will be up late grading) is really worth messing up my sleep that night. For me, it helps to cast things not just as prioritizing my sleep, but in terms of the importance of my training: "What's more important? The movie or my workout tomorrow? The gossipy conversation or recovering from that LSS run I did this morning?" When I put it in those terms, the answers are easy.

Diet. I will go into my views about diet in more detail in a subsequent chapter. Nevertheless, I have found that the amount and quality of food that I eat makes a big difference for my recovery. The closer I can get to the one gram of protein per pound of lean body weight standard, the better my recovery gets. I have also found that getting over "carbo-phobia" is very important for recovery, especially when I am in a base building or conditioning emphasis. When I don't eat those carbohydrates, I am generally more sluggish and less ready to go from day to day. There are probably as many of you reading this book who hamper your training by undereating as do by overeating. Where you are going to feel the effects of undereating most severely will be in your recovery. I also find that hydration really helps, too. I typically drink at least a gallon of water each day. I start the day with a quart of water and the juice from one lemon, and I drink a quart of water either during or immediately after my workout. I then find it easy to drink another half-gallon throughout the rest of the day.

Supplementation. I don't take a lot of supplements, and I never have. I'm not opposed to supplementation, and I don't think it's all a sham or any such thing. There are just very few supplements that have really moved the needle for me. I take a daily multi-vitamin to make sure I have all the basic nutrient boxes checked. I also include two servings of whey protein in my post-workout shake (along with one cup of berries and creatine). The shake, in particular, seems to keep me going strong post-workout, even after a pretty heavy beat down. The shake also helps me a lot in reaching my daily protein goal. As I just mentioned, I do take creatine monohydrate. I'm sure you don't need me to recount creatine's many performance-enhancing virtues. Trust that I have found them all to be true: I'm stronger, more muscular, and more explosive when I'm using creatine. I've also found that when I'm using creatine I can handle a greater volume of weight training, both within a single workout and across an entire week. Creatine is an important component of my recovery strategy.

Mobility Work. Before my workouts I do a 5-10 minute general warm-up (usually jogging or Airdyne) followed by some full-body dynamic stretching. Whether I am working out or not, I begin each day with about fifteen minutes of light mobility work. This consists of some bands, foam rolling, basic yoga, and dynamic stretching. I don't do anything particularly fancy, and I am not particularly regimented. I'll just get hooked on a few movements and then work them regularly for several weeks. This routine makes the biggest difference on my workout days off. By the end of a mostly sedentary day, I will feel pretty tight unless I have done some mobility work. I can really feel it in a workout following a day off when I have failed to do any mobility work. Frequently during the workday I will do 10-15 minutes of additional mobility work in my office, too. Following my conditioning workouts and BJJ training, I typically do about ten minutes of static stretching. During a recovery week I do an extended mobility session (20-30 minutes) following my grip/core/general conditioning/LSS workouts.

CENTRAL TAKE-AWAYS FROM CHAPTER 8

- Practice a policy of **preemptive action** regarding your recovery programming: don't passively wait for the problem to arise.

- Mandate **one non-negotiable day off** each week, and **one variable or flex day**.

- Implement a **3-1-3-1** block-level recovery plan.

- Adopt a simple **recovery routine** including practices for **sleep**, **diet**, **supplementation**, and **mobility work**.

CHAPTER 9:
PUTTING IT ALL TOGETHER

I have thrown a lot suggestions and ideas at you during the last several chapters. The emerging picture is probably far less complicated than it appears. In this chapter I am going to reproduce the training log I kept on the Tactical Barbell forum during the Fall of 2016. You will see how I implement all of the elements I have discussed: Operator I/A, conditioning, swings, BJJ, and the 3-1-3-1 recovery plan.

Some of the ideas discussed in this log will actually be taken up in detail in the following chapters when I introduce my thoughts on conditioning, testing, training maxes, and some specialized strength templates. So don't despair if some of these entries are a bit foreign.

This is my actual training log, transcribed daily from my notebook (I'm a bit of a dinosaur) with added commentary for the forum. It will give you some feel of the ups and downs of this sort of training. I only edited out questions and comments from other forum members and some of my own chatty asides. Feel free to join us for the full conversation:

http://tacticalbarbell.com/forum/index.php

You might find my notation a bit clumsy. For example, "SQ:310/3x5" means "Squat, 310lbs, three reps for five sets."

MON OCT 17

I'm starting a new block of Operator I/A. For the most part this will look a lot like plain old Black+Operator with 1-2 HIC (one E every 2nd week) and 1-2 Jiu-Jitsu practices each week. My cluster is SQ/OHP/WPU + DL every 3rd day. There will be times that I'll push the MS volume, and sometimes after a tough roll I'm not up for getting under the bar the next morning, so there will be some flex days. Some weeks might just be 1 HIC, and others might be 2. It depends on how I'm feeling. **Nothing**

really interesting is going to happen in this log, but I thought it might be useful to some of the people new to TB to see a more or less basic Operator block unfold.

To set this block up I did some "sort-of" maxing last week, mainly playing around with the 90% weights for what I was planning for my training maxes for one or two sets. That gives me a sense of how plausible those estimates are. I am playing with very conservative training maxes because I want a smooth series of forced progressions to keep me on a steady incline for the next several months. So here's last week:

Tuesday: jiu-jitsu -- pretty tough night!

Wednesday: I worked up to a very easy 315/3 on the SQ, and then did the 100 1H swings with the 48KG KB (in multiple sets).

Thursday: The Mound Street Hill (approx. 200 yards -- in my Apex videos I am running 1/2 of this hill) x 10

Friday: I worked up to 180/2 on the OHP and a very easy 405/5 on the DL. I haven't OHPed in a couple years, so I was really pleased with that double!

Saturday: LSS run/55 min (That was a very nice jaunt!)

Based on all that I moved my SQ T-max up a bit (I'm being conservative on the SQ, but that triple felt light; I could probably push those reps into the teens!), and I left DL and OHP maxes where I estimated them (I want to play conservatively on the DL, and aggressively on the OHP so the easy 5 and solid double were about right).

So finally, here is the first day of the new Block:

Operator I/A, Wave 1, Session 1/9 (75%)

SQ: 300/5x5

OHP: 135/5x5

WPU: BW+10/5x5

1H KB Swing: 40KG/50-30-20 (I took approx. 60 sec between these sets)

It occurred to me today between sets that I've never done the 40 KG for 100 consecutive swings, so I'd like to play with that goal. That first set of 50 was for real! Once that initial 50 gets relatively easy, I'll start compressing the break times until I'm doing two sets of 50. At that point I'll start subtracting reps from the second set and adding them to the first set.

Overall, this was a great first session of the block. I did OHP and WPU as "supersets," but I took at least 120 seconds rest for all the sets (OHP - 120 sec - WPU - 120 sec - OHP . . .). I felt as though I could go on banging out those fives on all three lifts indefinitely, which is how I want things during the 75% week. Crisp reps across the board and leave the gym hungry for your next session.

WED OCT 19

90 min of stand-up judo and ground work. There was a fair bit of full-speed situational drills and several rounds of live rolling. A pretty taxing session.

Today's action:

Operator I/A, Wave 1, Session 2/9

SQ: 300/5x5

OHP: 135/5x6

WPU: BW+10/5x6

Farmer Carry: 85lbs dumbells/up and down my alley (approx. 100 yds?) x 2

There are some points to be made about this session regarding auto regulation and weight room decision-making. I was feeling a bit south of awesome this morning after last night's hard work, so I expected just to hit the minimums and get out of the gym. In fact, I gave a second thought to "flexing" today. However, once I got under the bar, things were pretty snappy. I can't really make a call about how a session is going to go until I hit the first 1-2 working sets. This is important to remember when it comes to applying the "show up and put in the work principle." Just make a deal with yourself every day to do the minimums. Sometimes that is how it goes, and sometimes you will have a stellar workout.

Once I got going and started feeling great, I was actually very tempted to keep clipping out the 5s on the SQ, but I held off. I already have ten sets of SQ this week under my belt (which is really enough to have a pretty good week); I want to condition tomorrow; and I'm planning to SQ and DL on Friday, and maybe do Apex or Meat Eater this weekend. I've got a lot of work I want to get in over the next 72-96 hours, so restraint is the order of the day. Remember that the pertinent information for your weight room decisions is not only what is going on today, but what you want or need to do for the next several days. I'm not doing WPU on Friday, and I find that the stakes are always a bit lower on the upper body lifts, so I treated myself to an extra set of WPU and OHP.

OCT 20, 2016

Conditioning: Speed-Endurance Ladder x 1

This was a pretty standard conditioning day for me. I was up at 5:00, got my lemon water and coffee down, took some time to get my head right, and I was at the track by 6:00. I almost always do my conditioning (whether HIC, E, or GC) first thing in the morning, on an empty stomach. That's not for any really sophisticated reasons; I just feel better without something sloshing around in my gut, and my work day typically goes better when I get my workout finished very early in the day. When I lift, I prefer to go a bit later in the day (if I can, I try to do it during my lunch break). My back does better when I've been up and around for a few hours.

"SEL" is fast becoming one of my favorite drills; plenty of lung burn, but a bit easier to recover from than the hills. For similar reasons, I've become fond of "Anaerobic Capacity" too. I usually take "SEL" to two complete ladders, but I have a lot I want to do in the next 2-3 days, so one ladder was plenty. These are becoming my preferred drills to sandwich between tougher MS sessions.

FRI OCT 21

I actually enjoyed monkeying a bit with YouTube putting this together: https://www.youtube.com/watch?v=GYHxkR8ls_I

The video is the last sets of all of this:

Operator I/A, Wave 1, 3/9 (75%)

SQ: 300/5x4

OHP: 135/5x7

DL: 375/3x3

I felt great under the bar today, but I played it cool on the SQ because of the DLs on the horizon. I let it rip a bit on the OHP because I have nothing on the docket for the upper body until Monday. The DL is at 75% just like the other lifts, but since I'm still keep some serious swing volume, I'll be keeping the pulls to no more than triples. This is exactly how I want a day 3 of an OP week to go: I felt like I had mastered those weights, everything was snappy, and I'm looking forward to moving up to 80%. I felt the lack of the WPU, but that might be for the better; I tend to get some sore elbows from lots of pull-ups. We'll see how the DL mixes with my swing volume.

SAT OCT 22

Today's fun:

Apex: (sprint up + 2H swing 48KG x 10 + jog down) x 12

That was really fun. At 6:00 on a Saturday morning I just sprinted right up the middle of the street. Even after the DL yesterday, the swings felt great. I shut it down at 12 just to be cautious at the start of a new block. Interestingly, I haven't done Apex for quite a spell, but I have been doing a lot of plain hill sprints up a much longer hill (about twice the distance of my regular Apex hill). Normally, the sprinting part is harder for me, and the swings are easy. Today, I really had a much easier time with the sprints than usual. The extra sprint work might have paid off.

MONDAY, OCT 24

Operator I/A, Wave 1, 4/9 (80%)

SQ: 320/5x5

OHP: 145/5x5

WPU: BW+20/5x5

1H KB Swing: 40KB/50-30-20

This was a great Monday. I could've kept going on all three lifts, but I was happy with 5x5s across the board to start the week. When I used OP I/A last winter, I found that things went best for me when I hit about 10-13 sets of volume per lift/week (or in case of a "flex," a three day sequence at the same %), especially in the 70-85% range. Thus, if I can get five sets in on the first day of the week, I'm setting myself up to have a low-pressure situation to hit my sweet spot for the rest of the week. Even if I only hit the minimums on Wed and Fri, I'm still getting the volume I want, so the pressure is off as soon as I hit a good five on Monday. Thus, I tend to quit while I'm ahead when I hit that mark. The 100 swings with the 40KG KB were a lot easier this week. I took some video so I could get feedback on my swing form, but the glare from the sun in the background was really bad. I'll try again next week.

You might notice that I always lead with the SQ. There a few reasons for that. First, the SQ is always my highest priority lift. I find that the SQ is the key for my overall fitness. When I'm squatting well, everything seems to go right along with it. Second, I don't find that it tires me out for my other lifts. In fact, I find that I'm keyed in and pumped for the rest of the workout after my squats. This generally means I don't need to do as much warming up as I transition to my other exercises. Finally, I generally like to do the hardest task of the day first and then coast. This goes for everything in my life, not just pumping iron. Thus, I like to get those squats out of the way and then chill out and do some press'n and pull'n up.

TUE OCT 25

Tonight: 90 min of judo/jujitsu practice. Good session.

WED OCT 26

Operator I/A, Wave 1, 5/9 (80%)

SQ: 320/5x5

OHP: 145/5x5

WPU: BW+20/5x5

Farmer Carry: 85lbs dumbbells/100yd-ish x 2

Solid session. I actually felt good today after last night's hard practice. I'm now into double digits for the week for my total set volume for each exercise, so whatever I do Friday is in the "bonus round."

THU OCT 27

Hill sprints: "The Long Hill"/sprint up+jog down x 12 (no rests)

I'm planning to hit some LSS this weekend, so Apex is out for Saturday. I want to spend some time on the hills every week, and I don't want to do swings the day before I DL, so some regular hill sprints were the order for this morning. That hill is so long (180-200yds) that this workout feels a lot more like 200yd hill "resets" than traditional hill sprints. By the time I jog down, I'm feeling pretty well recovered. I really think this style of hill work has helped my game overall, so I'm keeping it in the mix.

FRI OCT 28

Operator I/A, Wave 1, 6/9 (80%)

https://www.youtube.com/watch?v=WtgniUDtv5w

SAT OCT 29

Standard Issue Fun Run + 15lbs vest/61 min

I did sub mountain climbers for the squats because there's been a lot of squatting in my very recent past.

MON OCT 31

OP I/A Wave 1 7/9 (85%)

SQ: 340/3x5

OHP: 155/3x5

WPU: BW+35/3x5

1-H KB Swing: 40KG/50-40-10

That was a lot of fun today. I had planned to cap the volume a bit more today, especially on the SQ, but the triples really kept coming. I had to tear myself away from the pull-up bar. I only stopped the OHP/WPU for the sake of time constraints. Things got a little long since I kept the breaks on the SQ closer to three minutes. I almost went for 60 continuous swings with the Bulldog, but I thought better of it. I did improve the second set to 40, so I'm progressing on that front.

TUE NOV 01

Tough Judo session tonight. I'm completely smoked. We'll see how the squats look in the morning.

WED NOV 02

Operator I/A Wave 1 8/9 (85%)

THU NOV 03

I went to a new BJJ class today. It was a great 90-min session: lots of drilling, and it ended with two 7-minute rounds of full-speed. With a 90% effort with the weights coming tomorrow or Saturday, I'm not going to add any additional conditioning.

FRI NOV 04

Operator I/A Wave 1 9/9 (90%)

Sat Nov 05

I went to a BJJ open mat this morning. I was planning just to have a light roll. Not so much, but it was very fun!

SUN NOV 06

600 meter resets x 6

WED NOV 09, 2016

Progressive Grip Circuit x 3

Quarterdeck Core x 5

This was just a little something to keep loose during my back-off. I started out with 35lb DB on the grip circuit, but by the third round I was down to 15lb DBs. This was an exercise in humility. It's a lot harder than it sounds. For QC I didn't add a vest and kept to minimums. The point was to get to a touch of movement.

THU NOV 10

I went to a lunch hour BJJ class. It was great session. I'm starting to get itchy to get back to the barbells next week.

FRI NOV 11

6.5 mile (approx.) run/54.28

I had wanted to ride my bike today, but it's the harvest here, so the roads are full of grain trucks. Not a great time to be flying down narrow country roads on a bike! There's no need to make another guy's already-hard job even more stressful because of my hobby.

Today was a real confirmation of the system. My last LSS was two weeks ago: a fun run. Before that it was three weeks since I did a real long distance run. That is, it's been nearly a month since I last ran any real distance. Nevertheless, today's run was really easy, but I was faster than usual on this route for an easy/casual run. I actually had to fight to keep my speed down a bit (I didn't want to turn this into a beatdown). I struggle with worrying that my endurance is going to crumble when I go "Black." I think it's because I'm a recovering fat person, and I fear that as soon as I back off the LSS I'm going to lose everything. That's bad thinking! A lot of people have the converse problem, i.e., "I'm going to lose all my strength when I go into my base building phase." The point of this system is that you don't need to train everything all at once in order to be decent at everything all at once. Once you get your tank full, you can maintain it very well with the occasional effort.

MON NOV 14

OP I/A Block 1, Wave 2, 1/9 (75%)

TUE NOV 15

Indoor Power Intervals on an Airdyne x 7.

Holy crap—that was a lot tougher than I expected it to be. I'm very impressed with the Airdyne after my first attempt to use this tool. I stayed on the bike for my rest interval but basically coasted. After the first sprint interval I seriously wanted to quit. I did all right with three minutes of rest, and the entire session (with a 5-min warm-up ride) came to 40 min. If you, like me, have injury/overuse issues that force you to moderate how much pounding you do on the hills/track, you will want to keep this workout in your toolbox.

WED NOV 16

OP I/A, Block 1, Wave 2, 2/9

SQ: 300/5x6

WPU: 10/5x6

OHP: 135/5x6

1H KB Swing: 88/70 - 30

I'm back on track. Everything felt very light and snappy. I got a little volume back in the SQ and OHP from what I missed on Monday. Getting 70 continuous 1-H swings with the "Bulldog" is a major bit of progress toward my goal of 100 continuous swings with that bell. I actually left a few in the tank on that first set! Notice that this is coming off a back-off week.

THU NOV 17

BJJ practice. We did three 7-minute (one-minute break) full speed matches at the end of practice. That was a great workout.

FRI NOV 18

OP I/A Block 1, Wave 2, 3/9 (75%)

Apex/48KG x 15 (sprint up, jog down, no rest, on my usual hill)

MON NOV 21

OP I/A, Block 1, Wave 2, 4/9 (80%)

TUE NOV 22

Indoor Power Intervals on the Airdyne x 7 (three minute-ish breaks)

That was easier than last week, but overall still a fairly unpleasant experience.

WED NOV 23

OP I/A, Block 1, Wave 2, 5/9 (80%)

5 mile run/35.20

FRI NOV 25

OP I/A, Block 1, Wave 2, 6/9 (80%)

SAT NOV 26

BJJ open mat. I rolled 4-5 matches, and I learned a lot and had a great workout.

MON NOV 28

OP I/A, Block 1, Wave 2, 6/9 (85%)

TUE NOV 29

Speed Endurance Ladder x 2

WED NOV 30

OP I/A, Block 1, Wave 1, 8/9 (85%)

SQ: 340/3x5

WPU: 35/3x5

OHP: 155/3x5

Just a small volume reduction and no extras. After a tough conditioning session yesterday, BJJ tomorrow, and 90% on Friday, I thought a little step back was in order.

On a related note, you might notice that I haven't been using the "Easy Week" principle, according to which you reduce your conditioning load by 50% during your heavy week of lifting. In most cases, the principle should be adhered to, but also note that I take a complete deload from lifting (and a deep reduction of conditioning) at the end of each three-week wave. If you schedule mandatory back-offs like that, you can get away with pushing the volume just a little bit.

THU DEC 01

BJJ -- lots of takedown work. Fun!

FRI DEC 02

OP I/A, Block 1, Wave 2, 9/9 (90%)

SQ: 360/3 x 3

WPU: 50/3x6

OHP: 165/3x5

DL: 400/3x2

There it is: a complete block of OP I/A. I left a lot of squats in the tank today since I wanted to give the DL some love. Regarding the DL, I'm in a holding pattern. If I can do a couple casual triples with 80% of a 500lb t-max, then I'm reasonably certain that I could pull it together and train up to a 550+ DL in a block or two. I'm happy having my DL right in that neighborhood.

I'm not quite sure about my next move. Next week is my mandatory back-off, but two weeks from tomorrow I have a BJJ tournament. I'm not sure whether it pays to start a new block until after the tournament.

SAT DEC 03

BJJ -- Open mat. I rolled three matches. It was a good workout.

So that's how a block of Operator I/A incorporating swings and working around BJJ can go for an ageless athlete. I came off this block feeling great. I increased my 3-rep max on overhead press and fell just short of an all-time PR on weighted pull-ups (that's about what I would expect, since I hadn't given either of those exercises much attention since before my summer base building phase). I didn't test my squat, for reasons we will discuss in "The Veteran War Horse Template" below. My bodyweight pull-up numbers were on point, and my run times were good for during continuation. I put on a touch of weight, but my body comp was better than ever. I had a small, lean gain.

I hope this chapter has helped to spell out for you how to put a lot of the principles we have discussed into concrete practice.

CHAPTER 10:
TRAINING MAXES AND TESTING

TRAINING MAXES:
HUMILITY FOR LONG-TERM PROGRESS

Using a training max is a practice wherein a trainee determines the weights for a strength program not based on 100% of his or her current one rep max but by some lesser percentage of his or her one rep max. Typically, a training max will be 90% of the trainee's true one rep max. For example, if your best bench press is 300lbs, your training max would be 270lbs. So, for the first week of Operator, for instance, you would do 3-5 x 5 with 190lbs (70% of your training max). This idea was made famous by Jim Wendler, and I recommend that you follow suit by putting it into practice in your own training.[28]

The obvious fact of the matter is that when using a training max, you are going to lift less weight than if you calculated your numbers based on 100% of your current one rep max. If our trainee had used his true one rep max, he would have started his first week bench pressing 210lbs, not the 190lbs he gets by using the 90% training max. Nobody much likes using a training max because everybody hates putting less weight on the bar. There is a fear that by moving less weight you will make less progress. The more weight I lift, the more strength gains I'll make, right? As we shall see, that's not always the case! There is also, let's be honest, some ego at stake. It's tough to realize that you could be squatting "three wheels" for reps in front of everyone in the gym if only you had used your true one rep max. As understandable as that attitude is, hopefully you are leaving immature, ego-driven thinking behind. Once again, think moderation. For any experienced lifter who has to balance strength against other fitness attributes and real life demands, a training max is the way to go for several reasons.

First, if you are using a high frequency program like Operator or Zulu (and I recommend that you do!), **you need to be able to come back and hit your numbers within 48-72 hours of your last workout**. These programs don't work like typical bodybuilding or some powerlifting schedules wherein you blast your legs or chest with both barrels but then have seven days until you need to be ready to perform those exercises again. Rather, with these programs, you need to be able to show up in the gym ready to perform each of your lifts 2-3 times each week. You don't have the luxury of a seven-day recovery between workouts. If you have "to grind" your way through your sets on day one, there is a good chance that things will be worse on Day 2, and by the time Day 3 rolls around, you are going to be lucky to get your work in. Thus, when playing the high frequency game, you need to give yourself a bit more room for recovery by employing a training max. This is obviously all the more important as we enter middle age and beyond.

Second, whatever kind of program you are on, **there are inevitably going to be days when you are not as sharp as you were back when you last tested your maxes**. For example, sometimes I'm squatting the day after an Apex session, but I would never test my squat the day after a tough hill workout. **We tend to test our maxes in nearly ideal recovery situations, but a lot of our training days are going to happen in less than ideal recovery situations because we have other priorities we are balancing.** If strength were your only priority, *maybe* you could get away without using a training max to determine your weights, but that's not the case for the ageless athlete who should be training across the fitness spectrum. Because you have so many mouths to feed you can't guarantee that you will be at your peak for every strength session. Thus, moderation demands that we work with a slightly reduced max to ensure you can get the work in.

Third, most of you reading this book probably determine your max not by actually performing a true max-effort single but by taking a rep max and using a formula to arrive at an estimated one rep max. That is all well and good, and in fact it is one of my preferred ways to test for anyone except a specialized strength athlete (see below), but you have to admit that you are now basing your program on a weight that you may never have actually lifted. There is a margin of error in even the most accurate estimating formula, so you need that margin of error reflected in your program. Err on the side of healthy skepticism by employing a training max.

Finally, as an ageless athlete, you need to give yourself a little more room to have a less than super day. The older trainee needs to optimize recovery, and he or she cannot expect optimal performance every day. Moreover, a lot of ageless athletes have been at the iron game for a long time, even several decades. If that is the case, you probably aren't only advanced in age, but also in the weights you are moving. Congratulations on that achievement, but know it comes at an expense. As you approach the absolute limits of your body's potential, your higher levels of performance are going to get costlier and harder to reproduce. You might not be able to match your most recent PR again on the drop of a hat, so it is unreasonable to expect that you can train based on that number day in and day out. Thus, **as we advance in years and/or the**

weights we are moving, it becomes even more important that we give ourselves a little wiggle room with a training max.

Does using a training max mean we will make less progress? Certainly not! Looking back, I have never said "That block would've been more productive if I hadn't used a training max," but I have seriously regretted not using one after I hit the wall and burned out. Don't fall in for silly, short-term thinking. What matters is progress in the long run. By using a training max, you will get more work of a higher quality under your belt over a longer stretch of time than if you trained at your absolute limit over the short term. Being able to come back again and again methodically is what makes for sustained lifelong progress. In short, by lifting a little less weight today, you will lift more tomorrow and well into the future.

That makes even more sense when you are using a high frequency program such as Operator. The key to this kind of training is the famous "greasing the groove" effect made popular by the renowned kettlebell and strength coach Pavel Tsatsouline. You are training your nervous system just as much as you are building muscle. **The point of high frequency programming is to develop skill at moving a certain amount of weight. You get under that weight and practice with it until you achieve technical perfection.** Once you have that down, you challenge your skillset by increasing the weight. Your goal should be that when 90-95% weeks come around, the barbells are still snapping right up. When you can crisply hit doubles at 95%, you know that you have gained significant strength. This approach might be boring and less impressive to onlookers, but it works. If you are serious about real results and not mere appearances, then it is hard to argue with it. **Forcing your ego out of the equation always rewards.**

If you want the magic of high frequency training, you need to work with numbers you can hit any day you show up in the gym, even a bad day. If you feel like you need more work, just push your volume a bit. The worst case scenario (short of getting hurt) is getting to Week 3, missing a bunch of marks, and realizing your whole block is botched. I strive to hit the golden mean of walking away from my workouts knowing that I really did get something done, while also feeling a little regret that I didn't do more. It's better to be a bit hungry.

Think of using a training max as another application of the Aristotelian conception of courage. Being brave certainly involves standing up to some threats, but it also involves making a careful retreat when that brings you closer to victory in the long run. Likewise, using less weight in your day-to-day training is not wimping out but doing what is more likely to bring you success in the long run. Getting crushed on Day 2 of your 95% week because you used an all-out, gut-busting PR to base your percentages on is not courageous. It's immoderate and stupid. The older you get, the less you can afford that sort of folly.

This point raises another advantage of using the training max: **it is stress free**. Your training should be a stress relief, or at least nothing that adds to your overall level of anxiety. For a lot of us this is recreation, and for those of you who need to do this professionally, fretting over your next workout is probably the last thing you need! If I know that some of the days in my 90-95% weeks are a little sketchy, I am going to worry a bit about that. If I know that I can hit my numbers come what may, I can walk into the gym with a completely carefree attitude. "De-stressing" your training (as we will discuss below) is also important for long-term persistence.

DETERMINING YOUR TRAINING MAX

So, how do you determine your training max? The most common rule of thumb is simply to use 90% of your current one rep max. For the most part 90% will do the trick, so it is a pretty good default practice. Another method is to use either your three rep max or two rep max instead of a one rep max. For example, if your last test on the overhead press was 200x3, you would then use 200 for your overhead press training max in your next block.

I don't use such a uniform approach. When I am setting up a strength block I put all six weeks into a spreadsheet that will calculate every day's numbers based on my training max. I start by setting 90% of my one rep max as my training max, and then I have a look at the numbers for all six weeks. If any day of the entire block looks the least questionable, I lower the training max. If there is any doubt that I can walk into the gym stressed out from work, with a head cold, a little sore from the previous day's sprints, and still smash my lifting numbers, then I lower the max. I repeat this process until I can look at every cell in the spreadsheet with complete confidence.

AGAINST GRATUITOUS RECREATIONAL TESTING

Testing your max, whether you do it by working to a true max effort single or by a rep max, is fun. Indeed, for those of us who are in this for entirely recreational purposes, testing might be the point of what we do in our strength training. What is more fun (in the gym at least!) than loading a big weight on a barbell and moving it yourself? Testing, however, is when you take your biggest injury risk and incur your greatest recovery expense. That's a worry for anybody, and for operational athletes who need to be physically good to go 24-7, those are downsides that need to be minimized. Moreover, testing can be particularly costly for the ageless athlete, especially those of you who are moving advanced or even elite weights. Right now for me a true, gut-busting, all-out max on the deadlift would leave me a mess for a week, however much fun it might be. Furthermore, if you test three or four of your lifts during your recovery week between blocks, there is some chance you will begin your next block with your CNS far from fully recharged. That means either an extra week off or starting your next block without full recovery. Either way, you hamper your progress. In short, you can ruin your whole recovery scheme by unnecessary testing.

My view is that you need to ask yourself whether you are **likely to learn something**

pertinent by testing. For a newbie, whose actual max is moving up at a steep curve, frequent testing (maybe even after a 6-week block) makes a lot of sense. When you start out, you initially make very big bounds of progress during your first several blocks of strength training, so the relationship between your training max and your actual one rep max can get way out of line in a hurry. Such a person is likely to learn something from the test that makes a difference for the next block because his or her max is probably increasing by leaps and bounds. Thus, I see nothing wrong with a relatively new lifter checking his or her true max every 1-2 blocks because by doing so such a trainee is likely to gain information that will make a significant change in how he or she sets up the next block of training. For example, the newbie can't rule out that he has made a twenty-five-pound jump in his squat max, and that is a very important datum for planning the next block.

Suppose that you are an experienced lifter whose progress curve is not nearly as steep anymore. How likely are you to learn something after just a six-week block? It's not very likely, in my experience. Right now, I'm pretty happy with even a 5-pound improvement on my overhead press max or a 1-rep improvement on my previous three-rep max in the deadlift. Do five pounds or one rep really make much difference for my next block? Probably not, especially because I'm going to be using a pretty conservative training max anyway. Most of the time I find testing to be a needless interruption in my training/recovery rhythm. Thus, **I prefer to use modest and methodical forced progressions for several blocks until I feel like I might learn something significant from a test**.

After having a few great blocks in a row such that the weights are really snapping up like you are doing "speed" work even during the 90-95% weeks, or when you have been forcing progression long enough that what used to be your doubles and triples are now your easy fives, then you are at the point when testing is likely to yield helpful information. Go ahead: pull the belt tight and have some fun finding a new max. **You earned the fun!** Just remember that you can get away with only so many of these really heavy days over your lifetime, so don't burn any of them unless you really think you have something to gain. Don't indulge in the excitement of testing until you have earned the privilege by putting in the daily work over the course of several solid blocks of training.

Unless you are actually competing in a strength sport, my advice is to avoid absolute, all-out max effort singles. These come at a great expense in terms of recovery and injury risk. Work to a rep max in the 3-6 rep range,[29] or follow the first of the two methods I will outline below should you prefer to work with singles.

TWO EFFICIENT WAYS TO TEST

I still don't like burning an "easy week" on testing, so my preferred method is what I call **testing within the block**. Following this method, you don't do your test during your recovery week after completing the block; instead, you build the tests into the last scheduled training day. There are two ways of doing this.

First, you can work up to some **singles within 95-100% of your <u>training max</u>** and gauge your progress based on how those singles feel. For example, suppose Smitty is using standard Operator with a 300lb training max for his bench press. Normally Smitty would then be scheduled to do 3-4 sets of 285x2 on the last day of the block. Smitty feels like he is due to check his progress on the bench press, so on the last day of the block he proceeds as follows:

Set 1: 285 (95%) x 2

Set 2: 285 (95%) x 2

Set 3: 295 (approx. 97.5%) x 1

If that last single is very easy and crisp after the first two doubles (and two days of 95% doubles earlier that week), Smitty has good reason to conclude that he is ready for a forced progression, and he hasn't had to burn any training/recovery days on testing. This workout might be a bit taxing, but if Smitty is using the 3-1-3-1 method, he has plenty of opportunity to recharge next week. Remember, Smitty could go all the way to 300lbs (100% of his training max) for his single. If you can handle your training max for an **easy single** at the end your workout, you are probably in a position to make a fairly aggressive forced progression. Maybe Smitty absolutely dominates 295 (97.5%). In that case, doing an additional single at 300lbs (100%) that day is fine. If you are leery of doing a heavy-ish single after the two doubles, then feel free just to work up to some singles in the 95-100% range and call it a day without doing the two doubles.

When employing this testing method, remember that **you are not going for an absolute one rep max**! You just want to get a feel for the weights at or near your current training max in order to gauge how aggressively to force progression (if at all). Don't turn this test into a disaster wherein you get pinned under 115% of your training max. **Never miss a rep!** I recommend this method only to a very seasoned trainee who can make sensible decisions in the gym and who knows how to gauge things by how the weights feel on any given day. That being said, this is my own preferred way of testing in most cases, but notice that it has taken me decades to get a feel for this sort of thing.

Another way to test within the block is to **do a rep max for the final set on the last 95% day.** In this case Smitty's bench press day might look like this:

Set 1: 285 (95%) x 2

Set 2: 285 (95%) x 2

Set 3: 285 (95%) x 6

As always, Smitty **stops short of failure on that last set**. If there is any question of whether you have another rep, then it is time to rack the barbell. Smitty can then put the information he gained into a max estimating formula to determine whether he needs to make a significant change in his training max. This rep max will cost you something, but hopefully you have some significant rest/recuperation planned for the coming week. Here, too, if you are leery of doing a rep max after the two heavy doubles, just work your way up to 95% for the rep max and call it a day without doing the two doubles first.

CENTRAL TAKE-AWAYS FROM CHAPTER 10

- Trainees using **high frequency programs, multi-dimensional athletes**, trainees **advanced** in age and/or lifting advanced weights, and trainees using **estimated maxes** should **all employ a training max**.

- However you determine your training max, **you should have complete confidence that you can complete every strength workout in your plan**.

- Only test when you have reason to conclude that you have something **significant to learn by checking your max**.

- Consider **testing within the block** by doing either a heavy-ish single >95% or a rep max on the last day of your strength block before a recovery week.

CHAPTER 11:
THE OLD WARHORSE TEMPLATE

A VICTIM OF YOUR OWN SUCCESS

I have a hypothesis that 90% isn't the same for everybody. The more advanced you are in terms of the weights you can handle, the costlier training near your limits will be. Admittedly, I have no real science to back that up. This is a hunch based on my own experiences and what I have seen happen to guys I have trained with over the years. Programming to account for this hunch has returned dividends for me.

For example, I don't think a 90% deadlift for a beginner/intermediate who is only pulling a max of 300 is going to have nearly the same consequences as a 90% pull for an advanced or elite guy pulling 600+. I'm not even convinced that the percentage of bodyweight being lifted is decisive, e.g., heavy training for a 600lbs deadlifter who weighs 280lbs is going to be costlier than the same for a new 140lb lifter with a deadlift max of 300lbs. The beginner/intermediate guy can go back to 270lbs fairly frequently and probably get away with it (in the short term!). Our advanced guy is going to get pummeled by playing close to 600lbs if he goes there with any regularity.

When I was powerlifting I was a lot heavier than I am now, and I was not worried very much about my maxes relative to my body weight. The absolute weights got big enough that I could only work at my heaviest levels for relatively short periods of time, **mostly just a few times each year** while I was peaking for a meet. If I played around my edge more frequently than that, I ran a pretty significant risk of burnout and injury. I found this to be particularly important when programming for the squat and deadlift, whereas I have always been able to get away with more for upper-body exercises. If you look at powerlifters who push the edge constantly, over the long haul they usually end up in some pretty sad shape orthopedically. The heavier the loads you move, the greater risk you incur, and the more crucial it will be to optimize recovery.

Part of my pet theory is that some of the problems that longtime trainees think are caused by aging are really just the fact that after training a couple decades they are now pushing advanced or even elite weights which are inherently costlier at any age. It's not necessarily your age that's hampering you but the consequences that inevitably come with the weight a seasoned warhorse can handle. You are probably a victim of your own success! This is something I discovered about myself while I was in my late twenties and early thirties—long before age was likely a factor. **The decisive factor isn't necessarily your calendar age but your training age**. You can get pretty "old" in the latter sense in a hurry once things start getting super heavy. Once again, this is solely based on my anectdotal experience, so take it with a grain of salt.

What if you are not a competitive powerlifter, or even someone who is moving advanced or elite weights? Should the ageless athlete in his or her forties and beyond take extra precautions? Assuming you are using a reasonable training max, then there is probably little reason to worry. If you are having no problems hitting your numbers every block; your joints are in good order; you are being disciplined in your recovery programming; and you aren't having injury or overtraining problems, then you are in the "If it ain't broke, then don't fix it!" category. Keep making good decisions, and keep on trucking. There is no need to impose limitations on your training in order to account for a problem you don't have, as long as you are playing it safely overall.

THE TRAINING MAX PROGRESSION TO A PEAK CYCLE

Suppose you are moving very heavy weights and subsequently feeling a bit battered. So how should a seasoned strength warhorse deal with this situation, if it arises? When it comes to the bench press, military press, and weighted pull-up, I haven't encountered much trouble, so I play those lifts just as I have discussed throughout this part of the book (more or less like any other Tactical Barbell athlete). I can play my pressing and weighted pull-ups fairly aggressively without any trouble. Where I need a little more programming subtlety is with the squat and the deadlift. Right now I could go out to my garage and squat >500lbs (>250% of my bodyweight) on a bar bet. Leaving aside my tendency to accept reckless dares, I know I could go 500+ safely with just a few weeks of peaking. If, however, I work in that vicinity very long, I will get hurt or burn out. So does that mean I can't make progress? Do I have to stay in perpetual maintenance mode? No. I just need a smarter, more long-term programming edge. If you struggle in a similar way with your upper body lifts, I believe the following approach will serve you well, too.

I typically do a very aggressive endurance phase during the summer months, and during that period I will barely touch a barbell. As you will see below, I tend to run my base building phase almost entirely with LSS (swimming, cycling, swimming, running), kettlebells, and calisthenics, but we won't digress on that topic here (see chapter 13 below). I usually come out of my endurance phase a little "skinny" and out of practice for my lifts. Thus, I want to muscle up a tad and need to practice my lifts quite a bit to get my strength skill back online. In short, when I start my continuation phase in the fall, it is time for high frequency and high volume, but not terribly high intensity. I also usually haven't done a lot of sprinting over the summer, so I want to get back on my horse with my favorite HIC workouts, such as Apex hill sprints and 600m resets.

So, I start my Black+Operator by setting a painfully low training max. This fall for the squat I started with 400lbs as my training max, which is a *pretty conservative* 80%. During that block I play aggressively with the volume. The weights are really pretty light, so this a great chance to grease the groove and build a little muscle with lots of sets. During a typical Operator week, I will try to get at least fifteen sets of squats, and sometimes more, during this block. This is a great time to work with Operator I/A.

At this point I will also push a little harder on the frequency and difficulty of my HIC. If my BJJ schedule permits, I will try to get three HIC during my typical week. Whatever frequency I can afford, during this block I will try to push the reps progressively on my hill sprints and other drills, trying to get to the advanced/operator levels. Since my lifting is relatively easy, I can usually get away with pushing a little hard on the hill and track. I will work in a LSS run, swim, or bike ride as needed. See my training log in chapter 9 for example of how this plays out in detail during the first block.

Assuming that the first block goes well, I then make a pretty aggressive forced progression for the second block, up to 5% of the current training max, depending on how things felt. For example, if at the end of an initial block of squats I was able to keep the volume high with snappy reps and good recovery throughout all six weeks, I will raise the training max for the next block by 5%, e.g., from 400 to 420. That's aggressive, but remember that I started with a conservative 80% training max. If you are following this program, then you are a veteran warhorse who can make a sound judgment.

In the second block, I pull back on the volume a bit for my lifts and HIC. Things are getting heavier, so you need to restrain other factors a bit. You can still do your HIC, even at the advanced/operator level, but you need to be attuned to how hard you are pushing and cut back when necessary. Check in with LSS sessions according to your continuation protocol. At the end of this block I will either force progression between 2-5%, or I will test within the block using one of the methods I outlined in the last chapter. Assuming all has gone well, and that I've gone with a 5% jump, I then move from 420 to 440 (rounding slightly).

The third block goes the same as the second: moderate volume with the barbells and HIC, but push a bit when you can. Work LSS in according to whatever continuation protocol you are following. At the end of the third block, I highly recommend that you do some sort of test and then adjust your training max accordingly.

Optimistically assuming 5% progressions all the way, I will start the fourth block with a 465lbs (rounding up a smidge) training max on the squat, which is 93% of my standard one rep squat max. I'm going to play a little aggressively with the intensity this block. If your test at the end of the third block is stellar, you might even push a 6-7% increase in the training max; just don't be reckless. Once again, this program is for wise veterans who can practice the Aristotelian virtue of courage.

Since you are pushing the intensity in the fourth block (things are finally getting heavy!), you are going to back off the volume a lot, both for your lifting and your HIC. For your 90-95% weeks you should plan to keep your sets and reps minimal, and that might go for the lighter weeks, too. Consider limiting your conditioning to just one HIC and maybe 1-2 easy (20-30 min) LSS each week. This block is about pure strength prioritization. Don't plan this for when you have a PT test or 10K race on the near horizon.

At the end of the fourth block, take a few days off and do a proper test. I recommend looking for a 3-5 rep PR with 100-107% of your training max for block four. That might be tough. **Have a spotter on hand!**

Once you finish block four (hopefully with a new PR in hand!), you can start the whole process over for another series of blocks beginning with an 80% training max (of your new 1RM), or you can go back into base building or a specialized template aimed at other goals.

Here are the nuts and bolts of this peaking cycle:

THE OLD WARHORSE TEMPLATE:
PROGRESSIVE TRAINING MAX PEAKING CYCLE

Block	Training Max	Lifting Volume	Conditioning Volume	Test?
1	80% training max based on PR from last continuation phase	High (5-10 sets) OP I/A %/Reps/sets recommended	Up to 3 HIC progressively pushing reps/intensity; E according to your continuation protocol	No
2	2-5% addition to the Block 1 training max (you can be a bit aggressive here)	Moderate (4-8 sets) OP I/A %/Reps/sets recommended	Up to 3 HIC each week; E according to your continuation protocol	Your choice
3	2-5% addition to Block 2 training max	Moderate (4-5 sets) Standard OP %/Reps/sets recommended	Up to 2 HIC each week; E according to your continuation protocol	Test within the block
4	2-5% addition (or even greater) to block 3 training max depending on your test result	Low (3-4 sets, minimal reps) Standard OP %/Reps/sets recommended	1 HIC (minimal intensity) and up to 2 easy LSS (20-30 min)	3 - r e p max with 100-107% t-max

Operator I/A is great for the first two blocks (when volume is high, but the weights are lighter), but you may want work closer to Standard Operator sets/reps/percentages for blocks three and four (heavier and lower volume). Don't be bashful about taking some "flex" days during those heavier blocks if you are having a hard time recovering.

If you are a Zulu guy or gal, go with I/A, but I recommend pushing the volume past the normal five-set limit during blocks 1 and 2 as I outline above (when you feel up to it!), as the weight will be relatively light. In blocks three and four, cap your sets as I outline above.

This cycle is a higher level manipulation aimed at bringing you to a peak over a longer sequence of blocks. If you would prefer to work with a longer or shorter peaking cycle, that is perfectly plausible; make any adjustments you want. If you are a seasoned warhorse who is feeling a bit battered, give this cycle a try during your next continuation phase, and you might surpass a long standing PR.

CENTRAL TAKE-AWAYS FROM CHAPTER 11

- Trainees lifting advanced or elite weights **may find it more difficult to train at the >90% intensity with any regularity**.

- **Unless you are experiencing this sort of problem**, continue with your currently effective plan.

- You can deal with this kind of problem by **progressively increasing your training max over a period of several blocks** until you are in a position to attempt a PR.

CHAPTER 12:
BACK "BREAK" TEMPLATES

PLAYING IT SAFELY WITH YOUR SPINE

If you have a back injury, then whether you squat or deadlift at all is something you need to decide in consultation with a physician. What I am about to discuss here is not any advice about how to deal with spinal injuries, how to rehabilitate such injuries, or even how to work around such injuries.

Even if you don't have serious back issues, occasionally you might want to construct a strength block that gives your back a little bit of a break. Although I tend to feel my best overall when I have high frequency squatting in the mix, I use this sort of truncated approach for a block here or there, just to give my body a little bit of a break from the heavier loads. I still train my lower body rigorously, but I cut down on the frequency a great deal. When I go this route, I only put one lower body barbell lift in my cluster (a squat variation or a deadlift variation), and I only perform that lift once per week. **This is not the best way to progress your squat or deadlift**, but it might be exactly the breather you need to stay in the game. Thus, if you are feeling a little creaky or beaten up from higher frequency squatting and/or deadlifting, then you might try one of these templates. When you are feeling like you are on your way to hitting the wall, going with one of these templates for your lower body lifts can prevent burnout.

THE SQUAT ONLY TEMPLATE

This won't be an easy template for your lower body; it's just lower frequency. We are going to put a little volume and intensity into a single day each week, but you will have a full seven days to recover and decompress after your squats. You will proceed per usual with your upper body lifts according to Operator or Zulu, but you will **squat only one day per week**. Whether you use Operator or Zulu, do your squats on the last day of the week. That way your heavier leg work will do the least to interfere with your upper-body lifts during the rest of the week. If you use the Operator I/A flex plan, just squat every second workout. Adjust as your conditioning and broader schedules demand. This also might be the time to push hard on the volume for your upper body lifts.

Your squat work will follow this progression:

> **Week 1**: work to your **best 6** for that day; **optional** 1-3 sets of 6 with 80% of your best 6
>
> **Week 2**: work to your **best 5** for that day; **optional** 1-3 sets of 5 with 85% of your best 5
>
> **Week 3**: work to your **best 3** for that day; **optional** 1-3 sets of 3 with 90% of your best 3

By "work up to your best 6" I mean that after you do your warm-ups, start performing progressively heavier sets of six until you reach what you think is **your best set for that day with absolutely perfect form and no risk of failure**. No psyching up, blaring death metal music, or partners slapping you with a power belt. This is your best "chill" set of six that you can hit that day. If there is the slightest doubt about whether you have another solid six in your tank, then shut it down for the day. Then do your down sets, if you are feeling up to it. You follow the same procedure for your best five and best three during the subsequent weeks. **You will go through two waves of this progression each block in order to match your regular Operator or Zulu progressions for your other exercises**.

I want you to work up to a top set for the day and then do some (optional) volume work instead of just using the Operator/Zulu sets/reps/percentages for that week because this is your only day squatting for the week. We want you to have a lots of time to recuperate your back, knees, and legs, but since you do have a lot of time to recuperate, you can push a little bit. Just keep it "chill" and have a little fun with this while also giving your body lots of room to recharge. **The back-off sets are optional.** Only do them when you are feeling really well, and there is no chance some extra work for your squat is going to interfere with anything else. If you have a day that you aren't "feeling the love," just call it quits with your best set of the day. Remember, it might take you several attempts to find your best set for the day, and you are supposed to be giving yourself a bit of a break. The extra down sets are not the hill to die in this program.

On two of your non-squatting days, you will do some **deadlift style accessories**. I recommend doing dumbbell Farmer Carries **and** kettlebell swings **or** Plank and Shank according the set/rep schemes we discussed in chapter 8 above. Certainly, these accessories are taxing to your lower body/back, but they don't carry near the loads as barbell lifts. Thus, we should exploit them as ways of giving the lower body attention while we are taking some time away from frequent heavy loading. An Operator week looks like this:

Day 1: BP/WPU + Dumbell Farmer Carry **and** KB Swings **or** Plank and Shank

Day 2: BP/WPU + Dumbell Farmer Carry **and** KB Swings **or** Plank and Shank

Day 3: BP/WPU/SQ to your best set (+ optional down sets)

When following an Operator I/A flex schedule, just do the accessories on your non-squatting days.

Here is the Zulu setup for this template:

Day 1: BP/WPU + Dumbell Farmer Carry **and** KB Swings **or** Plank and Shank

Day 2: OHP/Row

Day 3: BP/WPU+ Dumbell Farmer Carry **and** KB Swings **or** Plank and Shank

Day 4: OHP/Row/ SQ to your best set (+ optional down sets)

If you are concerned about doing swings/Plank and Shank the day before you squat, just leave them out on Day 3.

I don't see any reason to adjust your conditioning load when you are following this template. Since you are doing less squatting, you might, however, find that your legs are pretty fresh for your sprints.

THE DEADLIFT ONLY TEMPLATE

We only need to make some small tweaks to the deadlift for this template. First, we are going to cut down just a bit on the volume for the deadlift sets relative to what we did for the squat:

Week 1: work to your **best 5** for that day; **optional** 1-2 sets of 5 with 80% of your best 5

Week 2: work to your **best 4** for that day; **optional** 1-2 sets of 4 with 85% of your best 4

Week 3: work to your **best 3** for that day; **optional** 1-2 sets of 3 with 90% of your best 3

Secondly, we are going to change your accessories by using squatting-type exercises: the goblet, double kettlebell/dumbbell front squat, or pistol squats on your non-dead-lifting days. Operator would look like this:

Day 1: BP/WPU + Goblet Squats, Double KB FSQ, **or** Pistols 3 x 5-10

Day 2: BP/WPU + Goblet Squats, Double KB FSQ, **or** Pistols 3 x 5-10

Day 3: BP/WPU/DL to your best set (+ optional down sets)

Here is how Zulu looks with deadlift only:

Day 1: BP/WPU + Goblet Squats, Double KB FSQ, **or** Pistols 3 x 5-10

Day 2: OHP/Row

Day 3: OHP/Row + Goblet Squats, Double KB FSQ, **or** Pistols 3 x 5-10

Day 4: BP/WPU/SQ to your best set (+ optional down sets)

For the load on the accessories, just use good judgment. You probably aren't putting up much weight on these lifts, so there is room to do a few more reps. If you don't like doing squat accessories the day before you deadlift, then drop them from Day 3. You could also just make the pistol part of your main cluster for this block and program it as outlined in *Tactical Barbell*.[30]

CENTRAL TAKE-AWAYS FROM CHAPTER 12

- Occasional low frequency squatting or deadlifting can protect against burnout and other problems.

- Use either the **Squat Only Template** or the **Deadlift Only Template** and work to a best set of the day followed by some (optional) down sets for volume.

AGELESS ATHLETE PROFILE
FRED "DR. SQUAT" HATFIELD

There is no better example of an ageless strength athlete than Fred Hatfield. Famously known as "Dr. Squat" because of his impressive academic credentials and powerlifting feats, Hatfield has a long list of scholarly and athletic achievements to his name. Hatfield's most significant athletic feat occurred in 1987 when he "ATG" (ass-to-grass) squatted 1014 at a bodyweight of 255, wearing just wraps, a belt, and a single ply squat suit. Hatfield was one of the first powerlifters to break the ½ ton squat threshold, and **he did it at forty-five years old**. The 1000lbs squat has become common in elite powerlifting circles today, but Dr. Squat pulled this feat off before the age of Monolifts (he walked the squat out under his own power), triple-ply denim supportive gear, permissive "judging," and at a relatively low bodyweight compared to most of today's 1000lbs squatting monsters. It was a superhuman feat for an athlete at any stage of life!

PART 4:
CONDITIONING AND DIET FOR THE AGELESS ATHLETE

Reflect on what every project entails in both its initial and subsequent stages. Otherwise you will likely tackle it enthusiastically at first, since you haven't given thought to what comes next; but when things get difficult you'll wind up quitting the project in disgrace. You want to win at the Olympics? So do I—who doesn't? It's a glorious achievement; but reflect on what's entailed both now and later on before committing to it. You have to submit to discipline, maintain a strict diet, abstain from rich foods, exercise under compulsion at set times in weather hot and cold, refrain from drinking water or wine whenever you want—in short, you have to hand yourself over to your trainer as if he were your doctor.

Epictetus, Enchiridion[31]

CHAPTER 13:
AGELESS ATHLETE BASE BUILDING

DON'T BE AFRAID TO TAKE A BREAK FROM HEAVY BARBELLS

One of the distinct marks of the Tactical Barbell system is the emphasis on aerobic endurance as part of an overall, multi-domain approach to fitness. Aerobic development has been much maligned in recent years, with short, intense, anaerobic workouts taking center stage in a lot of popular fitness programs. A high level of anaerobic work capacity, as important as it is, is just one component of what it takes to be an overall well-conditioned human being. Part of that puzzle is also aerobic endurance.[32] For the ageless athlete, aerobic conditioning is particularly important due to its benefits for cardiovascular health, mood, and weight control. Since it can be very difficult to advance both maximum strength and aerobic endurance simultaneously—especially since endurance training can be easily overdone—the best approach is to let these different attributes take front and center (while others are deemphasized) during separate training phases.

The standard Tactical Barbell base building approach comes as an eight-week block. In the first five weeks the trainee focuses exclusively on aerobic endurance (think LSS running) and strength endurance (no heavy weights!). In the final three weeks, limited max strength work and HIC are reintroduced, and pure endurance is backed off a bit.[33]

Many of you reading this probably panic at the thought of not touching a heavily loaded barbell for five weeks (followed by three weeks of limited barbell work). Does that mean I will lose all my gains on my maxes? Before you despair completely, note that there is K. Black's "Strength First" option, according to which you keep max strength for the first five weeks of base building and emphasize strength endurance only for the final three weeks.[34]

That being said, I encourage ageless athletes to avoid the Strength First option. First, you will lose far less on your maxes during base building than you think. Sleuth around the Tactical Barbell forum and subreddit, and you will find posts from **trainees who took the standard approach and actually gained strength!** Even if you do lose strength, that loss will be minor and temporary. It might take you a few weeks to get your strength skills back to where they were at the end of your last continuation phase, but everything will indeed return. In fact, often you will experience a rebound effect: after having a break from the stress of heavy lifting for an extended period, your body actually makes gains beyond where you left off once you reintroduce maximum strength stimulus. **I typically leave heavy barbell work out the mix for ten to twelve weeks during the summer while I work on endurance**. My muscularity and max strength are down a bit at the end of that phase, but as soon as I get back into continuation I get a nice rebound on both attributes. This sort of ebb and flow is the cost of doing business for a multi-domain athlete. You might need to suffer through some very small ups and downs if you are going to balance all the priorities you need to address. The downside, however, has been greatly exaggerated! Once again, restraint is part of the ideal of moderation.

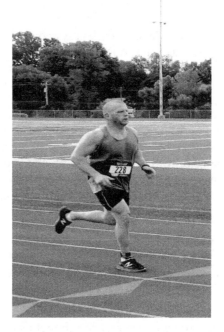

This is literally the final few steps of my base building last summer after nearly three months of no heavy lifting!

Second, stepping away from the barbells for several weeks actually has long term advantages in addition to making room for developing other attributes. Heavy lifting, even when done properly and programmed efficiently, is going to produce some wear and tear on your body. Operational athletes and ageless athletes in general need to guard against chronic overuse injuries. Giving your body a break from the grind of heavy squat/bench press/deadlift/overhead press should be part of your annual plan. Your joints, ligaments, and nervous system will benefit greatly from an extended recharge, and that will only contribute to your long term progress. As we discussed earlier, this sort of extended break from demanding exercises is one of the keys for the ageless athlete.

Finally, one of the biggest psychological hurdles for the ageless athlete is boredom and stagnation. If you don't have a PT test right around the corner that your job rides on, sooner or later motivation is going to flag. A couple months dedicated to radically different goals and styles of training can help pull you out of a rut. If you are going to keep this up for decades, some variety is necessary to keep your interest. I personally enjoy spending the summer months outdoors chugging away on endurance activities, which refreshes me to get back to the weights in the fall.

APPLYING THE MINIMAL EFFECTIVE DOSE TO BASE BUILDING FOR THE AGELESS ATHLETE

There are some tweaks to the standard base building approach that the ageless athlete should consider. As written in *TB2*, the standard base building template peaks at a required 3 x 60 minute (at least!) LSS sessions in a single week, and gives you the option to add an additional endurance session on Recovery Day. However, **we recommend that in typical cases ageless athletes limit themselves to no more than 3 x 30 minute LSS sessions per week during base building.** For the average trainee who just wants to build a sound aerobic base without pushing toward high-level endurance goals, any more endurance work than that is going to cut into other valued attributes (strength and muscularity will be particularly threatened). **For most ageless athletes, 3 x 30 minute sessions are the minimally effective dose.**

Thus, **Ageless Athlete Base Building** is as follows:

Day	Week	Week 2	Week 3	Week 4
1	Tango Circuit x 2	Tango Circuit x 3	Tango Circuit x 3 (compress rest interval)	Tango Circuit x 4
2	LSS x 30 min	LSS x 30 min	LSS x 30 min	LSS x 30 min
3	LSS x 30 min	LSS x 30 min	LSS x 30 min	LSS x 30 min
4	Tango Circuit x 2	Tango Circuit x 3	Tango Circuit x 3 (compress rest intervals)	Tango Circuit x 4
5	Recovery	Recovery	Recovery	Recovery
6	LSS x 30 min	LSS x 30 min	LSS x 30 min	LSS x 30 min
7	Off	Off	Off	Off

Day	Week 5	Week 6	Week 7	Week 8
1	Tango Circuit x 4 (compress rest intervals)	Max Strength	Max Strength	Max Strength
2	LSS x 30 min	HIC	HIC	HIC
3	LSS x 30 min	Recovery	Recovery	Recovery
4	Tango Circuit x 4 (compress rest intervals)	Max Strength	Max Strength	Max Strength
5	Recovery	HIC	HIC	HIC
6	LSS x 30 min	LSS x 30	LSS x 30	LSS x 30
7	Off	Off	Off	Off

Weeks 1-5 are straight forward enough: simply work your way through the thirty-minute LSS sessions and Tango Circuits. If you want more work, you can add some additional trips through your strength endurance circuit on your recovery day or add some light recreational sports. Just make sure that recovery day stays "easy." During Week 3 and Week 5 instead of adding rounds to your Tango Circuit you will try to finish faster than last week by compressing your rest intervals between exercises/rounds. If you don't like LSS running two days in a row, feel free to switch Days 3 and 4. Be careful with that measure, as many of you will find that the Tango Circuits leave you sore for a day or two (especially when you start compressing the rest intervals).

I prefer Tango Circuits to Alpha or Bravo Circuits for recreational athletes. The latter are probably better for progressing your push-ups, pull-ups, sit-ups, etc., but if you aren't under a lot of pressure to push your calisthenics numbers for your job, you will find Tango a challenging and more manageable way to get a few weeks of solid strength endurance work under your belt.[35] If you prefer Bravo, or you need to start with Alpha, switch things as you like.

I cannot stress enough the importance of taking these five weeks to focus on strength endurance circuits for the ageless athletes. The point is not just improving your strength endurance (though that is not a bad thing). Rather, the real benefit for the ageless athlete is the general physical preparedness effect this sort of training causes. Several weeks of gently strengthening the muscles and ligaments while giving the joints and nervous system a chance to recover from heavy lifting is going to help sustain good orthopedic health over the long haul and contribute to a nice strength and muscle rebound after base building. You will also find that Tango Circuits leave you huffing and puffing, so they can help boost your metabolism. These workouts tend to be brief, which will give you a chance to put a little extra time into your mobility work. I have found that a moderate Tango Circuit followed by some static stretching are just what the doctor ordered the morning after a tough BJJ practice.

Weeks 6-8 proceed exactly as prescribed in the standard base building template in *TB2*, with the exception of the thirty-minute cap on all LSS sessions.[36]

If you are out to do more than "check the box" on your aerobic endurance, e.g., you are an endurance athlete, a tactical athlete with a job that requires more endurance, or you simply like the challenge of extended endurance workouts, then by all means do more. As you will see below, I definitely fall in the category of those who like endurance challenges. Notice, however, that anything more than the minimally effective dose will come at some expense to your other attributes. There are always costs to be weighed against benefits, especially for the ageless athlete.

CENTRAL TAKE-AWAYS FROM CHAPTER 13

- Take the opportunity to use the first five weeks of base building to **give your body a break** from the strain of heavy barbell lifting while reaping the benefits of **Tango Circuits**.

- Your default base building approach should be the **Ageless Athlete Base Building, which limits LSS to 3 x 30 per week**.

CHAPTER 14:
TWO NOVEL BASE BUILDING APPLICATIONS

MY SUMMER BASE BUILDING PHASE

When in doubt, use Ageless Athlete Base Building! You will stock your endurance reserves, recharge your nervous system and joints, and come back refreshed and motivated to hammer the weights and sprints. There is no need to overcomplicate this when you have an effective approach in hand. That being said, I don't have an entirely conventional approach to base building. In fact, you might not call it "base building" at all; it's more of a heavy endurance training phase. In this section, I will highlight some of my tweaks that you can take or leave.

First, I stay in my endurance phase for ten to twelve weeks, rather than the standard eight-week block. As I divulged earlier, I'm a bit of an endurance junky, so I like to get all of that out of my system for the year during the summer while the weather is nice. I realize that this extended endurance phase might cost me something in terms of my strength development, but I have some strength to burn, and I really love spending those long hours outdoors during the summer.

Second, I mix up my endurance activities quite a bit. I love distance running, and if I had my way, that would be the lion's share of my endurance mileage. The problem, however, is that I have found that long distance running is probably the costliest drain on my recovery resources. Moreover, I have to watch my total running volume because otherwise I will start to get trouble with my Achilles tendons. As I say, "My Achilles tendon is my Achilles heel."

The need to moderate my running mileage during my endurance phase has led me to take up swimming and cycling. My first foray into cycling actually occurred one summer when I had seriously strained my Achilles tendon and couldn't do much on my feet for six weeks. I had previously hated riding a bike, but that summer I fell in love with cycling. Now I include cycling in my conditioning mix both for LSS and HIC. Sprints on a road bike are much harder than you might think! I also transport myself in daily life almost exclusively on my bike. That extra activity in my daily routine helps keep me relatively lean.

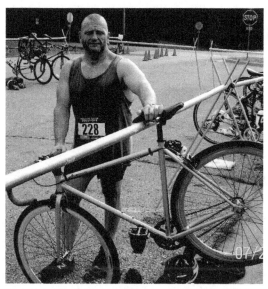

I completed a sprint triathlon on a single speed road bike. I was able to cover a hilly, twelve-mile cycling route in just over thirty-six minutes.

I am not by any stretch of the imagination a natural swimmer. I have never particularly liked the water, and until mid-life I could barely swim to save my life. Ironically, my kids are all very good competitive swimmers. Watching them develop in the pool led me to realize that swimming is a noble athletic endeavor. Thus, using my kids as instructors, I took it up. Things initially progressed pretty slowly. At first I couldn't complete a single lap of freestyle! I had no buoyancy; I just sank like a stone and had to keep moving to stay afloat. It took over a year of persistent practice (and several very disturbing moments for the lifeguards at my local YMCA!), but I got to the point where I can casually swim 1600m (32 laps) continuously. I'm very slow, and I doubt that swimming will ever be a particularly strong part of my game. Nevertheless, swimming gives me a great conditioning option (for both LSS and HIC) that is very joint-friendly and helpful when working around the weather (I use an indoor pool).

Maybe more importantly, swimming has done much to improve me psychologically. Initially I had a lot of anxiety in the water. During my first couple months of swimming, I had a lot of workouts that ended with me nearly panicking as I choked on a lung full of water. Learning to calm down, not to worry about anything but my current stroke, and simply to put the work in were key steps toward my becoming a competent swimmer. Developing that attitude is crucial for lifelong progress as an athlete (and maybe much more).

As I mentioned earlier, I don't do much maximum strength work during my endurance phase. On my non-LSS days, I tend to work with kettlebells, calisthenics, various weighted carries, weighted stair climbing, or barbell complexes. I do a lot of workouts very similar to the Tango Circuits.[37] Frankly I don't really have much of a structuring principle at all for my strength work during this phase. I approach it with a spirit of play. If there is a bodyweight feat I want to play around with (muscle-ups, handstand push-ups, pistols, gymnastics rings, etc.), I work on that. Maybe I want to do a circuit of kettlebell exercises; that's fine too. Last summer I seriously got into rope/pegboard climbing. Occasionally I'll throw in something like Apex Hill Sprints just to challenge myself. This is my chance to play without worrying about measuring up to a rigorously defined program. Usually by the end of the summer I'm ready to get back to serious business aimed at definite goals, but early on I enjoy the latitude to experiment. There is no doubt that results-oriented, meticulously planned training protocols are the way to go in the long term. That doesn't mean, however, you can't go out and play around in the short term once you have built a solid strength foundation.

Unless you are a very experienced and disciplined athlete, I recommend that you stay on a carefully planned program year-round. Ironically, it takes a lot self-knowledge and discipline to play like a kid.

Here is what a typical week of my endurance phase looks like:

Sunday: Off

Monday: 6-9 mile LSS run

Tuesday: BJJ

Wednesday: Strength: circuits, calisthenics, climbing, etc.

Thursday: 1600m swim

Friday: Strength: circuits, calisthenics, climbing, etc.

Saturday: 15-30 mile cycling or a 10K Fun Run

If I train BJJ more than once or I throw in a HIC workout, I will drop one of the strength days or do a light strength session that same day. I adhere very strictly to the Tactical Barbell II "talk test" for my running/swimming/cycling. Especially on my running, slowing my pace has been crucial for long term progress. I used to think that a good run required that I need a bucket at the end. That attitude led to burn-out, frustration, and injury. I started to see the problem, and I slowed my LSS running pace to 9 min/mile, and everything got better. The distance I was covering increased, and when I decided to go faster it was easier. The distance on the run on any given day just depends on how I'm feeling, the route (hills?), and the weather. The same goes for the cycling. The swim usually comes in at 1600m of combined freestyle and breast-stroke. Since I have a day off on Sunday, I do tend to challenge myself on my Saturday ride. Sometimes I'll do a challenging cycling-running "brick" or a swimming-running combination.

About once every month I will do a long Fun Run on Saturday. One of my training partners and I used to do an endurance challenge on the weekends. Frequently it was something like an 800m swim followed by 10K LSS run, but eventually we started playing around with the fun runs. We began with K. Black's "Standard Issue" going out to 10K using the basic calisthenics (alternating between 10 burpees and 20 push-ups/20 squats every six minutes for the duration of the run). We worked up to a grueling 8-mile run using K. Black's advanced calisthenics (10 burpees, 50 squats, *and* 30 push-ups every six minutes for the entire duration of the run). We also experimented with some of our own variations. For example, one weekend we did a 7.5-mile run (that included running up a 2-mile steady incline) around a circuit of ten playgrounds. At each playground we did 10 pull-ups, 25 feet-elevated push-ups, and 10 toes-to-bar leg raises. These workouts made for a really exciting weekly challenge. They also check the strength endurance box too. I find that all of my aerobic endurance, anaerobic work capacity, and strength endurance measures peak when I have fun runs in my regular mix. Get creative and use all your local resources when constructing your own fun runs. I can't vouch for my heart rate at all points during a fun run, so be careful with this option when running a strict aerobic endurance base building block.

Notice that the schedule I follow during the summers involves much more in the way of endurance work than is recommended in Ageless Athlete Base Building. In order to build a decent aerobic base, as we discussed in the last section, there is no need for anything more 3 x 30 minute LSS sessions each week during an eight-week base building phase. I do much more than that because I enjoy endurance activities and occasionally competing in endurance sports. I also have very little problem rebuilding muscle and strength during my continuation phase, so I'm comfortable absorbing the costs of my LSS habit. If you don't particularly care for endurance challenges or you are a "hardgainer" who has a hard time gaining and/or keeping strength and muscle, this is probably not an approach for you.

This style of training is not good enough to prepare you for a serious triathlon. For that you will need a specialized program. It did, however, get me well prepped for my first sprint triathlon, so if you are planning for a shorter event you might give this a try. The point of all this is that as you gain experience about what works for you, there is a lot of room to build your own distinctive approach while remaining **broadly** within the parameters of the Tactical Barbell system. Base building in particular lends itself to your own innovations. **You simply need to get out on the road and put the work in.** The way you do that is largely up to you.

USING A BASE BUILDING APPROACH TO START FROM GROUND ZERO

By the summer of 2014 my wife, Jennifer, could barely walk around the block. She was suffering terrible back pain from an arthritic disc, which forced her to be more or less sedentary for three years since our youngest child was born. Jennifer hit rock bottom in terms of fitness that winter. She was forty-three years old, had been through multiple C-sections, broken her femur earlier in life (which gives her some trouble), had a very painful back, and all sorts of real life demands on her time. Jennifer had every available excuse to throw in the towel on her fitness, and nobody would have blamed her for doing so. At that point, however, rather than giving up, Jennifer decided to take control of the situation. Keep that in mind when analyzing your own self-serving biases! Jennifer is probably the toughest athlete in our house.

She began working with her physician and physical therapist to address the back pain. They put her on a gradual program of progressive stretching and anti-inflammatory medication. If you or someone you love is facing serious orthopedic difficulties, **start with the medical professionals**. Once you have that squared away, you can begin worrying about fitness achievements per the directions of your doctors. Jennifer had repeatedly tried to change in the past, but her efforts met mostly with frustration. Only when she got the flexibility/mobility piece of the puzzle in place was Jennifer ready to make any further fitness progress. **First step: get back on your feet**.

That got the ball rolling, and after a couple months her doctors gave her the O.K. for more strenuous exercise—no small achievement. She started a regime of yoga, Pilates, and calisthenics. After a few months of that regime she had built a pretty good base of mobility, strength, and strength endurance. Jennifer was more or less pain free and feeling optimistic about her fitness for the first time in years.

Deciding on her next move posed a puzzle. Previously, Jennifer had been involved in rock climbing, competed in powerlifting, trained with kettlebells, and completed triathlons. Because of her back, despite its improvement, kettlebells and barbells were strictly "no go." She couldn't handle those modalities pain-free. As far as triathlons go, she loved swimming and cycling but really hated the running. The problem is that both swimming and cycling also tended to tweak Jen's back a bit when done in any extensive measure. That left running, something Jennifer has always disliked, and she always thought of herself as a bad runner. She was committed to getting a high level of fitness, so she took on the challenge of facing her greatest athletic weakness. Who was imposing this limitation on her running but herself?[38] She set the goal of being able to compete in a 5K race.

So how do you program running for a middle-aged trainee, who is not by disposition a runner, and who isn't in terribly good aerobic condition? It was a real struggle at first. Jennifer would go out and push hard, but that usually ended up pretty miserably. Every running session she would have certain distance or time marks she wanted to meet, which led to a lot of stress. There was no lack of frustration during the summer of 2015, but she did achieve her goal of running a 5K race that September. Good: we established that Jen can do this, even if the programming wasn't quite right.

That winter she went back into her strength focus (yoga, Pilates, calisthenics) with some occasional running. In the spring of 2016, we decided to adopt something like the Tactical Barbell base building approach for Jen's running. She would just go out and chug along at a moderate pace (observing the talk test) for as long as she felt like she could handle it on as many days each week as she felt like running. There was no pressure to cover any distance. Just put the work in casually, and come home when you feel like it. If you feel good-to-go tomorrow, go out again. If not, have a rest.

The results were incredible! By the end of the summer, **Jennifer could run continuously for over an hour.** She was forty-five years old, and that is something she had never achieved before. She had a distance PR of just over five miles, which was also a lifetime best. She could handle a running load of four sessions each week. It was no longer a question of whether she could complete a 5K, but how fast she could do it. Her times in that race had also reached all-time bests. Not surprisingly, Jennifer's other fitness markers greatly improved. For example, with her newfound aerobic base, she was able to introduce some pretty heavy-duty HIC sessions into her regular regime (400m resets and hill sprints), something she had never done before.

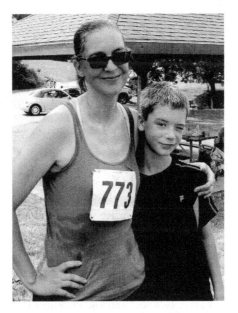

Who says you can't? Here is Jennifer after completing the running portion of a team triathlon she did with some of our children.

Here is what a typical training week looked like for Jennifer in the summer of 2016:

Sunday: Hill sprints x 10 or 400m resets x 4

Monday: LSS run (20-30 min)

Tuesday: Strength circuit + 20 min LSS (elliptical trainer)

Wednesday: LSS run (30-45 min)

Thursday: Strength circuit + 20 min LSS (elliptical trainer) **or** OFF

Friday: LSS run (45-60 min – Challenge Day)

Saturday: Off

That schedule was the peak volume of Jennifer's program for the summer, but since then she has settled into 2 x 20-30 minute LSS runs, 1 x HIC (hill sprints/resets), and two strength endurance or yoga sessions each week. During the summer she may try to push out past the 60 minute mark again, bur for the most part Jennifer now stays in the parameters of Ageless Athlete Base Building.

Jennifer would be the first person to tell you that her running is not impressive in terms of the distances she covers or the time it takes her to do it. She isn't going to be running in Boston in April anytime soon. That's fine, but her case is instructive in two ways. First, it's a great example of overcoming self-imposed limitations. Jennifer had sold herself short for years regarding what she could achieve as a runner. Second, it's a great example of what base building can do for you. This approach was integral for Jennifer's getting to the point where she can live a runner's lifestyle and enjoy all the physical and psychological benefits that come along with it. If taking the time to build a solid aerobic base can do this for a forty-five-year-old mother of six with an arthritic back, then what can it do for you?

CENTRAL TAKE-AWAYS FROM CHAPTER 14

- The ageless athlete should stay ahead of overuse problems by employing **a variety of endurances activities**.

- An experienced and disciplined athlete can **use base building as an opportunity to reload** by approaching strength work with a playful attitude.

- For anyone wanting to build (or rebuild) fitness from the ground up, **aerobic base building is the best place to begin**.

CHAPTER 15:
APEX HILL SPRINTS, DUKU-DUKU, AND HIC INTENSITY

PROGRESSING APEX HILL SPRINTS

Since *Tactical Barbell II* was released in the summer of 2015, Apex Hill Sprints have become an obsession for many of us. By now most of you reading this book are probably familiar with this gem. For those new to Tactical Barbell, Apex is a coupling of hill sprints and kettlebell swings. It's a match made in Heaven (or Hell!) if ever there was one. You run up the hill, knock out ten two-handed swings, and repeat as many times as you can handle. It's just that easy...well, maybe "easy" is not the best way to put it. I was impressed with the simplicity and comprehensive benefits of this drill: strength, speed, anaerobic capacity, and mental toughness are all addressed. I immediately put it in my training mix with the goal of reaching Black's "Advanced/Operator" standard: 15+ rounds using the 48KG kettlebell ("The Beast") with no breaks and jogging down the hill.

I have been running hill sprints since I started training for football in junior high (and yes, at the time Ronald Reagan was the President of the United States, and we were still listening to music on cassette tapes). I've also been swinging kettlebells for about ten years. I started Apex in July of 2015 with a 70lb bell and quickly got to twenty rounds jogging down and no breaks. By November I was hitting fifteen rounds with The Beast, and one day in February I pushed it all the way to twenty. Here are some highlights from a fifteen-round Apex workout:

https://www.youtube.com/watch?v=-U6BDJDshoo&edit=vd

Progress at Apex can be tricky, especially when you are just starting out. Here is a fictional, though typical, case:

Smitty wants to progress at Apex. He has a hill nearby and a 24KG kettlebell. He is a dedicated and disciplined trainee, so he hits the hill 2-3 times every week. The only problem is that after about five trips, even with some breaks and walking down the slope, Smitty is completely wasted and looking for a bucket. Now he seems to be stuck, and he is not seeing improvements. In fact, he is getting a bit discouraged and burnt out.

I have three recommendations for Smitty: (a) Build your aerobic base, (b) master your kettlebell, and (c) approach your Apex programming with a "periodized" mindset. Let's look at each of these recommendations in some detail.

(a) *Build your aerobic base*. Sure, Apex is a paradigmatic HIC-style workout. There is, however, a considerable endurance aspect to this sort of training. For example, when I go twenty rounds, I am going to be on my feet continuously for 30+ minutes. Somebody who cannot easily sustain a 40+ minute LSS run is going to wilt very quickly when he tries to push his Apex rounds into the double digits. Like everything else in TB programing, becoming awesome begins with building your base. Once your body gets used to sustained periods of work, everything gets easier. Thus, my first recommendation for Smitty is to make sure he is getting his endurance tank topped off with a solid 8-12 week annual base building block.

(b) *Master your kettlebell*. I had long since become very adept at swinging The Beast before I ever tried Apex. I could do 100 1-handed swings with the 48KG in 4.30 (1:1 work to rest), so ten 1-handed swings even after a hill sprint were really the "easy part" for me. In fact, sometimes I feel as though I recover a bit from the hill sprint while I am doing the ten swings. The point is that your progress on the Apex will move along faster once you have really mastered your kettlebell. I highly recommend you incorporate one of the kettlebell swing protocols that I have outlined earlier into your regular plan, or take time out to do a specialized kettlebell program. You will find the carryover to Apex is tremendous.

(c) *Approach your Apex programming with a "periodized" mindset*. When you go to the gym and squat or bench press, you don't expect to hit a 100% 1RM every time out. As any reader of TB knows, that is the path to ruin. Rather, you spend most of your time in the 70-90% range. You vary the intensity of your work through that range, and rarely do you absolutely redline the engine. In my experience, Apex behaves much more like barbell training than other forms of HIC. I have zero science to back that up (so help yourself to disagree), but that is definitely my experience.

What this amounts to practically for me is to incorporate variations in either volume (the number of rounds) or intensity (the length of the sprint) in my Apex sessions. Notice that I don't vary the weight of the kettlebell because I use only a bell that I have mastered. The swings are sort of a "given." I tend toward volume variations. My PR on my preferred hill (the one I'm running in the videos) is twenty trips, but most days I do 15 rounds. If I don't feel like "Super Jim" or there's a big squat on the horizon, I might settle for 12 rounds. If I want to push myself a bit, I'll go to 17 rounds. Notice that I'm keeping it in 60-85% effort range (in terms of volume). In any event, I almost always leave the hill feeling like I have a couple rounds left in the proverbial tank.

What this means for our guy Smitty is that that he might need to settle for some fairly short sessions. If his PR is 5 rounds, then most days he should keep his sessions to 3-4 rounds. He won't be pushing to near vomiting every session. If he doesn't feel like he is getting enough work in, he can always add some more sessions. Lower volume, higher frequency, crisp sessions…sound familiar? If Smitty absolutely cannot stand such a brief workout, there is nothing stopping him from adding some burpees or a fast 800-1600m run as a finisher, but I would prefer high frequency, high quality before adding anything on top of Apex. Nobody ever became a fat slob by doing hill sprints + swings at 80% three times weekly.

You could also lower the "intensity" (in terms of the length of hill) and raise the volume by increasing the number of rounds. In this case, Smitty might run only half the length of his hill (or just find a shorter hill) but push the number of reps. For example, by sprinting half the distance Smitty might make as many 8-10 rounds. Once again, the idea is to keep the average total effort at a manageable 75-85%.

Here's how we might put it all together into a mini-cycle:

Week 1 – Distance emphasis: full hill for 60-90% of PR number of rounds

Week 2 – Repetition emphasis: 1/2 the distance for as many reps to reach 75-90% perceived exertion

Smitty can run three of these mini-cycles right along with an Operator or Zulu template, and then at the end of a six week (or longer) block he can test his Apex progress just like his barbell lifts. On test day let it rip! Smart money says that Smitty will have a new max on Apex, and he can adjust his numbers for the next block accordingly.

The question of frequency for your Apex sessions is likely to arise. Like any frequency/recovery issue the "right answer" is going to vary among athletes depending on age, diet, other stressors, experience, the weight of the kettlebell, difficulty of the hill, etc. For me, one Apex session each week is enough. Knocking out 150-200 swings with The Beast is definitely going to cost you something in terms of recovery, especially for middle-aged trainees. See our earlier discussion of programming for kettlebell swings for an outline of a training week that involves Apex. Younger trainees or those using light kettlebells are probably going to get away with a bit more.

There are other variables you can tinker with: jogging versus walking down the hill, and the duration (if any) of the rest period at the bottom. The grade of the slope is another factor you can play with, assuming you have multiple hills available. Suffice it to say that these recommendations are not the last word on making Apex progress, and you can come up with a very effective way of managing the load by manipu-lating any of these variables. Whatever you come up with, just remember that all-out, go-till-you-puke training is not a long-term recipe for progress. It is the very antithesis of the ideal of moderation we are pursuing. There is a time and a place for pushing your limits (save the "death wish" intensity for test day), but the bulk of your work needs to be in that not-as-exciting but effective sweet spot. Moderate the difficulty of your Apex sessions so that you can show up at your hill and methodically put in the work. Over time the effects of all those swings and all those trips up and down will accumulate, and you will find yourself making big progress.

For those of you who struggle more with the hill sprint than the swing, consider incorporating a longer hill to use for basic hill sprints. Recently I took a break from swinging, and I just focused on standard hill sprints, but on a longer hill. My normal hill (the one in the video) is about 100m, but that is only half the distance up that particular slope. I started running 8-12 complete trips up that hill (approx. 200m) twice weekly. After about eight weeks I transitioned back to Apex, and I found that I was much more comfortable in the 15-17 round range than before. The "shorter" sprints just seemed easier now.

NEVER AGAIN: THE DUKU-DUKU CHALLENGE

Duku-Duku (a.k.a. Praetorian Hills) is a challenge session from Tactical Barbell II. This probably isn't something you are going to do on a weekly or even monthly basis. In fact, I have done it twice, and I'm in no hurry to try it again! It is in fact a pretty reckless and stupid thing to do. I guess we all have our moments. I get a lot of questions on how to progress on this challenge, so I'll give you my thoughts along those lines.

Duku-Duku begins with five kettlebell goblet squats at the bottom of the hill. You then, without putting the kettlebell down, run up the hill. Once on top, without putting the kettlebell down, you do ten swings. You then walk down the hill and repeat, but as soon as you put the kettlebell down, you are finished for the day. Ideally you will get to five rounds with your kettlebell.

The first time I tried Duku-Duku, I used a 55lbs kettlebell, and I did twelve rounds. I actually thought that doing twenty Apex sprints with The Beast was much harder. I tried Duku-Duku several months later, but this time I used the 48KG. I completed five rounds, but **that was hands down the hardest single exercise I have ever done**. I was pretty miserable when I finished it. Here is a video of the entire ordeal:

https://www.youtube.com/watch?v=K0nFMmFQPus

I didn't do anything in particular to prepare for this challenge. In fact, I think the best preparation for Duku-Duku is Apex Hill Sprints. Here, too, mastering your kettlebell is key: the swings were actually a recovery opportunity after the hard carry up the hill. My grip was also very well-adapted to handling The Beast. At the end of the challenge, my legs were smoked as though I had done a 20-rep squat workout from hell, so I suspect having a solid squatting base is likewise important.

The point here is that meeting this challenge (or any challenge of this nature) is really a matter of developing excellent overall fitness. The way you do that is simply by implementing the sort of multi-dimensional programming we have been discussing throughout this book. Follow your regular protocols, and these sorts of challenges will take care of themselves. It goes without saying that the ageless athlete should make challenge sessions pretty few and far between. Occasionally throw down the gauntlet, but choose your battles wisely because it will come at an expense. If, by the way, you ever try Duku-Duku with The Beast, don't make plans for the rest of the day!

SOME THOUGHTS ON HIC INTENSITY FOR AGELESS ATHLETES

I have frequently seen middle-aged trainees wonder whether they should run their sprints at 100% max effort, or whether they should moderate their pace to avoid injury. I have found that, given my Achilles woes, I need to moderate a bit.

First of all, I always begin a HIC session with a good warmup. I start with some dynamic stretching, focusing on the hamstrings, hips, and calves, with some upper-body work, too. I also jog for 800m or five minutes. After that I will often do 2-3 easy (building to about 80% effort) sprints of about 50m. I warm up until I feel ready to go. Suppose I am running 400m sprints for my workout, with the plan of doing six rounds. On my first round I will consciously keep the pace to about 90%. That's enough to get me huffing and puffing. If I feel well and nothing is tight or nagging me, then I start to increase the pace each round, trying to beat my time on the previous lap. At about two rounds into the workout I will be able to tell what kind of day I'm having and how hard or long I can push myself. By the time I get to rounds 4-5 I'm usually right around my best time for that distance. I will struggle to stay there for the remainder of the workout. If at any time I start to feel the slightest twinge of trouble, I will moderate the pace or shut it down for the day. I use a similar method for all my sprinting workouts, e.g., the first rep or two of hill sprints will be very hard efforts, but they are also diagnostic to see what I can handle that day.

You can push your HIC very hard, even maximal effort, but you need to be careful. Take the time to get a proper warmup, and build slowly throughout your workout. If things aren't going well, live to fight another day. Once again, part of courage is knowing when to back away from a fight.

CENTRAL TAKE-AWAYS FROM CHAPTER 15

- Progress at Apex Hill Sprints by **building your aerobic base, mastering your kettlebell**, and **applying periodization principles**.

- Prepare for challenge sessions, such as Duku-Duku, by having **a solid overall training plan that produces multi-domain fitness**.

- The ageless athlete can push HIC very hard, but **you need to warm up and patiently gauge your limits for the day**.

CHAPTER 16:
SOME DIET STRATEGIES

I'm probably the last guy who should be throwing around diet advice. As you can see in the pictures and videos in this book, I'm not a fitness model. I've never checked my body fat percentage, but I know it's not 4%. Far from it! Thus, if you are looking for advice on getting completely shredded, you will need to look elsewhere. I haven't walked that path, so I have no advice to give.

I have, however, managed to lose about 100lbs and to keep it off for over ten years. As I like to put it, I'm a former fat person who is pretty far down the road to recovery. That path requires constant vigilance, so I do give my diet some thought. I have also successfully managed to eat to perform well in my workouts and competitions. When it comes to eating in order to stay reasonably lean over the long haul and to able to train hard, I can offer some advice.

DO I HAVE TO COUNT CALORIES?

For some reason, diet is a touchy topic. Few points of disagreement get fitness people more worked up than how to eat right. (Whether to wear a weightlifting belt is tied with the whole concept of CrossFit for a close second place.) One of the primary controversies surrounding diet is whether you need to count calories or meticulously weigh your portions in order to make progress. Like a typical professor of philosophy, I am going to answer this question with "Yes and no."

I suspect that if you want to get to a single digit body fat percentage, then you are going to need to get very precise. You will probably need to count and weigh things very accurately. Likewise, if you are trying to lose weight, ultimately you will need to burn more than you eat. Having at least a rough sense of your calories consumed versus your calories burned is going to be helpful. If you are trying only to fuel your workouts and more or less maintain your current weight or body composition, then you can probably manage portions intuitively and be fine.

After bulking up for my last powerlifting meet in 2013 I wanted to lose a good bit of weight. My approach was to start with a food journal. I wrote down everything I ate for two weeks and then carefully analyzed the log. I began by cutting out foods that were just plain stupid and left my diet otherwise unchanged. **Step one: Quit eating like you have a death wish.** I dropped some weight that way very quickly, but eventually things plateaued. I kept a food journal again for two weeks. Once again I looked where I could make some cuts, and the weight started coming off again. I repeated this process periodically until I reached my goal (down to 188lbs from 238lbs).

The periodic food journaling approach worked to help me lose weight immediately, but more importantly it gave me a lot of self-knowledge. It showed me exactly what I need to eat to lose weight, gain muscle, or maintain while performing at a high level. Whenever I talk to someone about losing weight, I always advise them to take this approach in the beginning. This doesn't mean you need to log every meal for the rest of your life. I haven't done so in a couple years. Once you build good intuitions about what works for your diet, you don't need the hassle anymore. An initial period of regular logging will help you gain those intuitions.

ROUTINE IS KING

I have followed the same basic eating plan for the last three years almost religiously. I found a set of foods and an eating schedule that really works for me, so I adhere to it very strictly. There are occasional small tweaks and bumps in the road, but the main elements remain the same. Preparing these meals has become second nature for me. Packing my day's meals before going to work is just as routine as brushing my teeth.

Is this routine boring? Sure, at times. But that is part of the price. Do I eat foods I like all the time? No, not always. I eat tuna every day, and I really don't have a natural taste for it. The routine helps with that. Once you have been sticking with something for a couple years, you can get used to just about anything. I strongly encourage you to establish a workable eating routine as your first dietary priority.

Your best routine is probably based on a lot of idiosyncratic factors. Nevertheless, here is my typical food day. This is an example of my day when I work out over my lunch break:

> 6:00 AM: 4 whole eggs, two slices of organic toast, fresh squeezed lemon juice, 1 quart of water
>
> 9:00 AM: 1 cup of plain Greek yogurt, spinach (sometimes a piece of fruit)
>
> 11:00 AM: Pre-workout: tablespoon of chia seeds, 1 piece of fruit
>
> 12:30 PM: Post-workout shake: 2 scoops of whey protein, 5g of creatine monohydrate, 1 cup of frozen berries

2:00 PM: 1 turkey burger, spinach, whole wheat crackers or brown rice

4:00 PM: 5oz of tuna, a whole green pepper, handful of almonds

6:00 PM: Whatever the family has for dinner, usually a lean meat and a lot of veggies

There is nothing earth-shattering in this meal plan. It's your basic "eat several small meals, each more or less balanced with macronutrients," approach. If I feel like I want to get more protein, I might add a scoop of whey protein in the evening or another serving of Greek yogurt. On Friday nights I have a cheat meal consisting of whatever I want. This isn't innovative, but it does show that I have found a list of foods and a schedule for eating them that has kept me performing very well for years. It now only takes me ten minutes to put this all together in the morning, and I don't need to think twice about what I am going to eat throughout the day. I don't recommend that you necessarily copy this diet (though you could do worse) but that you look for a list of foods and a schedule that you can work into a locked-down routine. That is the long term key.

Another benefit of following a definite routine is that it lets me think less about food. As a recovering fat body, I can get a little obsessive about my diet and bodyweight or composition. I could very easily go down an OCD rabbit hole worrying about what and how much I'm eating. By having an eating routine that I follow like a zombie, I am less tempted to fall into that anxiety pit. Keeping to a proven routine keeps me from constantly worry about whether I'm getting the diet piece right. I know this routine works well for me because I have years of success behind it, so I trust it.

Finally, a word about alcohol. You will notice in my food routine that there is no alcohol mentioned. Occasionally I will have a couple beers with my cheat meal on a Friday night, and I will have a couple drinks on major holidays or social events. I'm no teetotaler, but in my late thirties I started to notice some ill effects from relatively moderate consumption of alcohol. Anything more than just 1-2 beers was followed by lowered motivation, depressed moods, and poor sleep for a couple days. I took this as a sign that I needed to moderate my consumption rigorously. In fact, alcohol was one of the first things I cut out entirely when I started losing weight. There are a lot of other variables, but there is a pretty significant correlation for me between extremely moderate consumption of alcohol (sometimes complete abstinence) and better performance, mood, and body composition. I write this not to preach to anyone but to note that your alcohol consumption might be something you need to keep a close eye on as you strive for high levels of fitness into middle age and beyond.

CENTRAL TAKE-AWAYS FROM CHAPTER 16

- Though you might need to count calories to get shredded, you can get yourself on the path to a reasonable body composition and performance level with **a temporary food journaling** approach.

- The key to long-term dietary success is establishing an **eating routine** that works for you.

- Consider **seriously moderating alcohol consumption**.

AGELESS ATHLETE PROFILE
BARBARA BUDER

If you troll around the internet you can find a legion of examples of ultra endurance athletes killing it into their sixties, seventies, and eighties. For my money, they are all heroic, but among the most impressive is Sister Madonna Buder. That's right: she is a Roman Catholic nun, and she didn't take up running until she was forty-eight years old. **Sister Madonna has since completed FORTY-FIVE IRONMAN TRIATHLONS.** She single-handedly forced the Ironman organization to add competitive categories for the 75-79 and the 80-84 age groups. The good sister's motto? "The only failure is not to try because your effort in itself is a success."[39]

PART 5:
PERSISTENCE

Every habit and faculty is formed or strengthened by the corresponding act—walking makes you walk better, running makes you a better runner. If you want to be literate, read; if you want to be a painter, paint.

Epictetus, Discourses[40]

CHAPTER 17:
DISCIPLINE

EMOTIONAL INTENSITY: A RECIPE FOR FAILURE

If you belong to a commercial gym, every January you spend half of your workout time waiting for your turn on the squat rack because there are so many fresh, highly motivated faces around trying to make good on their New Year's resolutions. Sadly, the majority of the new gym members won't pull it off. By the end of January they are starting to dwindle, and by the summer you mostly see only the old hands that have been hanging around for years.[41] It doesn't matter how well you construct your fitness program if you don't execute it. Persistence is the most important factor in achieving a high level of fitness. There is plenty of good information available for free on the Internet about how to train, eat, and recover. There is no lack of places to exercise; whatever you can afford, you can still run in the street and do calisthenics. Everybody has the time. One hundred burpees every morning for the next year would get you a long way down the path. No, the biggest thing standing between people and fitness is actually "pulling the trigger" on a fitness plan and sticking to it.

People typically start a fitness regime all fired up. They are motivated by the new possibilities, and they throw themselves into their program with gusto. They eat, sleep, drink, and breathe it. It's all about intensity and emotion. "This time I'm going to make it happen by working harder than all the other times I quit!" Sound familiar? What's also familiar is that they typically quit fairly soon.

The problem is that **emotional intensity is not a good long term strategy to be successful at anything.** I don't care if it is a fitness program, obtaining a graduate degree, or completing a military selection course (I'm told), being fired up is not going to deliver you in the end. The reason is that emotional intensity is inevitably going to ebb and flow. You can't count on it to be there when you really need it.

Sooner or later, your emotions are going to fail you, and there will be a day when you don't "feel the love" for your run, the hours you need to put in at the library, or whatever challenge your drill sergeant throws at you. As an ageless athlete, you know well that you don't have endless stores of youthful enthusiasm. **If all you have in your psychological arsenal is emotional intensity, then you will fail**.

The reliance on emotional intensity is why most people beginning fitness programs are going to fail. There will be days you don't want to do it. There will be weeks, even months, when you don't have the feelings and the passion. Very few nights will you be excited about going to bed at 9:00PM (so that you can be in the gym at 5:30 the next morning). If all you have are your feelings, the first time your buddies invite you out for beers you will bail on your workout in the morning. It is similar to a romantic relationship. It can start out fueled by intense emotions, and this might keep it going pretty strong for a while. When the initial romantic fervor cools, you will go your separate ways unless there is some deeper foundation.

WHAT I LEARNED MAXING MY SQUAT EVERYDAY

What else do you need besides emotional intensity? **Discipline. A disciplined person is someone who can control himself or herself. He or she can hold to a pattern of behavior, whatever his or her emotional dispositions**. Notice that a disciplined person isn't necessarily fired up, or even particularly enthusiastic. **He or she is in control** and sticks to the pattern. He or she doesn't need continuous emotional charges to stay on task.

A concrete example from my own training will help illustrate discipline and its value. For most of my training history, Squat Day was something I would get fired up for. Imagine a pot of coffee, grinding heavy metal music, and training partners screaming. The only way I was going to get through it was on pure adrenaline—emotional intensity. This worked for a while, and even a pretty long while, but it wasn't ultimately sustainable, and it certainly wasn't something I could summon every day of the week.

A few winters back I gave an Eastern-Bloc inspired high frequency squatting program a try. The idea was to work up to squatting to a max single every weekday, Monday through Friday. By max here, the idea is not a gut-busting, one-rep PR effort. Rather, the plan was just to work up to the best single you could handle that day **without any kind of psyching up**. What is the best you can do without drawing on your emotional intensity? Show up in the gym, hit your best completely relaxed single for the day, and then go home. If you have a great day, congrats. If you have a bad day, that's fine because you will be back tomorrow to do it again. Every day was completely business-like. I had to keep my emotions in complete check because getting fired up every day was going to deplete my adrenaline pretty quickly. It was like squatting with Mr. Spock from *Star Trek*.

This sounded like heresy to me, but I gave it a try. I just showed up every day and did my single. I mostly trained alone. I walked in the gym, warmed-up, worked up to my best "chill" effort for the day, and moved on. A lot of the days I listened to the morning news on NPR while squatting. That was a far cry from my adrenaline-pumping power-lifting days! There were some really terrible mornings when I had to call it quits at 350x1, and there were fun streaks when I would consistently cut through singles in the high 400's several days on end. I eventually got to the point where I was squatting five days every week, and by the end of the winter I casually hit a lifetime bodyweight relative PR of 500lbs while weighing 190.[42]

What's the point? My earlier practice was all about emotional intensity, whereas my high frequency squatting project was an application of discipline. My squat workouts were not about being fired up and intense but about showing up and putting the work in. **I didn't have high expectations for any day in particular**. Some days were going to be good, and some were going to be bad. Since I was getting under the bar every day, I had to let myself have bad days. By lowering my daily expectations (and allowing myself to have bad days), I ultimately ended up getting more work done. I was squatting five days each week!

If I had thought I had to perform at my best and squat 95% every day, there is no way I could've handled the pressure. I would have had to psyche myself up constantly, and sooner or later (probably sooner!) I would have failed miserably. Rather, **squatting became a habit**. I didn't have to give it much thought. Squatting a "max" single was just how I started my day. It wasn't something I psyched up for any more than the other parts of my daily routine.

That is the difference between discipline and emotional intensity. Discipline is not concerned with short term emotional satisfaction but with long term results. Discipline is a consistent pattern of behavior that is followed independently of emotional intensity. In short, **discipline is a habit**.

If you want to persist, then training has to become second nature in much the same way that brushing your teeth is second nature. You don't have to make a daily decision to brush your teeth. It's just what you do. It is almost in your subconscious pattern of behavior. That is where I am now with my workouts, and that's what I find in most people who are successful ageless athletes: **their training is almost completely habitual**. It is not a question of whether I will train on a given day. What I will do, how hard I will go, what adjustments have to made, etc. are often in question. But training *as such* isn't a question. It is a habit.

Being disciplined isn't some magical act of will. Disciplined people are not magicians or spiritual masters. Hardly. They just have impeccable habits. Disciplined people may have deep and powerful emotional reserves they can draw on when they need it, but that is not how they get through the daily grind necessary for success. There are no emotional conjuring tricks that will keep you on your program. In fact, the more you rely on emotional mojo, the more you are setting yourself up for failure. You need to get beyond emotional intensity and into the solid realm of discipline.

SO HOW DO I GET DISCIPLINE?

If you think of it, this question raises a serious problem. How do you make yourself become disciplined, when you aren't already disciplined? To obtain discipline, you need to persist and build good habits. But how can you persist and build habits if you aren't in some sense disciplined already? It seems we have a circular problem on our hands: to become disciplined, I need to build certain habits, but to build those habits, I need to be disciplined.

Aristotle really wrestled with this problem. Here is how he put his solution: "the virtues we get by first exercising them, as also happens in the case of the arts as well. For the things we have to learn before we can do them, we learn by doing them, e.g. men become builders by building and lyre players by playing the lyre; so too we become just by doing just acts, temperate by doing temperate acts, brave by doing brave acts."[43] In other words, **you basically have to go through the motions**. As Aristotle says it, the only thing that will give you the virtue of justice is to practice doing acts of justice, in the same way that you learn any other complicated pattern of behavior, e.g., carpentry or playing a musical instrument. You don't have to like being a just person when you first start out; in fact, you probably won't like it very much at all. You merely have to go through the motions of justice, and over the long term (maybe most of your life) you will get the taste for it, and eventually it will become second nature. If your acting justly is only a matter of how you feel, then you will fall back into being unjust as soon as you don't feel like being fair. Once again, emotional intensity doesn't sustain anything.

If you have children, this will probably make a lot of sense to you. When children are young, you mostly can't explain to them why they need to be fair or temperate. All you can do is make them do fair and temperate actions, and eventually they will get the habit. You can't begin with what they feel like doing. They won't like the right things at first. Far from it! Occasionally, they might get excited about living up to your expectations, but those feelings are mostly short-lived. Eventually, however, with enough practice they will get the hang of it and even start to like it, once the practice becomes a habit.[44]

The same thing goes for your training. You don't have to like it initially. You don't have to act like you have a habit you don't have yet. You just need to show up. That's all you have to do on any given day. Just show up in the gym, at the track, in the pool, etc. Commit to doing only the least necessary to start. That's all you need to do. **Discipline is an acquired taste.** If you really aren't feeling up to it, commit to doing just half of your scheduled workout. Just show up—without any promises to yourself that your workout is going to be awesome. **Your workout doesn't have to be awesome to be effective. Your workout only needs to happen to be effective**.

Paradoxically, if you have trouble persisting in your training, **I want you to lower your expectations for the short term**. I don't mean that you should lower your expectations for what you can achieve in the long term—hardly. Much of what I have written is aimed to make the opposite point. Rather, I mean that you may need to lower your expectations for what you are going to do today. When you tell yourself that you are going to smash your PR everyday "come hell or high water," and you don't live up to that expectation day in and day out, you are learning to fail. You are constantly dealing with frustration. Of course, people quit when they train with this attitude because nobody can live up to those sorts of expectations in the long run. The only expectation you need to live up is to go through the motions.

These lower (short term!) expectations are going to lower your anxieties about training and make it easier to persist. You will then put the work in, and you will build the habit. You will become disciplined. The intense, fired up, "balls to the wall" days will be there—lots of 'em! Just don't try to plan one for every workout because that simply isn't going to happen.

Finally, a word about stress. You're busy; I don't doubt that. That's probably true of everybody but tenured college professors. You have a lot of pressures on you professionally and from your family. Those certainly have to come first—before your training. Don't, however, make your training into a bigger stressor than it needs to be. If you feel as though you need to show up every day and "kill it" at the gym, you are going to feel some pressure to perform. Your training will be one more expectation you need to live up to in your life. Eventually, you will fail to meet that unreasonable expectation, which is going to increase the anxiety and stress associated with your training. Don't do that to yourself, especially if you want to persist in your program. You don't need to "kill it" every day. You just need to go through the motions. Lower your expectations, and that will lower your stress. Your training should be a stress release, so just let it happen. By lowering your expectations for each workout, you will de-stress your training, and I bet your chances to persist will increase.

"YOU JUST GOTTA FINISH SEAN!"

The need to achieve discipline through a short term lowering of expectations is not a worry for rank newbies alone. Take the example of Sean, a former student and training partner of mine. We used to work out together while he was an under-graduate college student trying to get a spot in BUDS with the USN after graduating. Sean grew up in the water playing water polo and surfing. He is a great athlete: strong as an ox, pumps out endless pull-ups, and swims like a dolphin.

Sean's only problem when we first started training together was that his running was bad. No joke. I'm not a world-class runner, but initially Sean couldn't hang with me in any distance greater than a 5K. He could crush me in sprints and shorter distances, but his aerobic endurance was in pretty poor condition. He was pretty much all sprints in the pool, too. The first time we went out for a 10K together, Sean vomited a jalapeño cheeseburger about four miles into the route. (He also needed to improve his pre-workout nutrition strategy.) Every time we went for a run the same series of events occurred: Sean would see that he was off the pace he needed to be able to reach his long term goals, and he would try to solve his problem by pure effort. He would push his pace too hard and then crash and burn. This went on for weeks.

Finally, one day before our run I dared Sean to take his watch off. No timing; just hang with me at my slow "old man" pace. I also told him to remind himself constantly that "You just gotta finish Sean!" That became my mantra to him throughout the run. "Don't worry about how you are doing. Don't worry about what you need to be able to do two years from now. Just keep putting one foot in front of the other and cover today's distance." That day we ran eight miles, an all-time distance PR for Sean. Things took off from there. On one of his last days training here, Sean ran thirteen miles, cycled fifteen miles, and swam 1600m. His swimming, calisthenics, and running numbers were all good enough to earn a BUDS contract.[45]

Renouncing emotional intensity, lowering short term expectations, and focusing on developing discipline (in place of emotional intensity) were crucial for the progress of even a well-developed athlete in his prime like Sean.

CENTRAL TAKE-AWAYS FROM CHAPTER 17

- Most people fail to persist in training programs because they rely on **emotional intensity**.

- Persistence is possible only through **discipline**, and discipline is primarily a **habit**.

- Begin the process of becoming disciplined by **lowering your short term expectations** so you can **go through the motions** until you build the right habits.

CHAPTER 18:
GUARDING AGAINST DOING TOO MUCH

GOOD INTRA-WORKOUT DECISION MAKING

Much of what we discussed in the last chapter was aimed at how to avoid doing too little. "How do I manage to work out at all when I don't feel like doing it?" That is certainly a problem for many trainees (or soon-to-be former trainees). I suspect, however, that many of you reading this book are like myself and really have the opposite problem: "How do I keep from doing too much when I feel like Superman?" That is, if you are like me, your failure of moderation in working out is more on the side of excess, not deficiency. As we have discussed, doing too much is probably a bigger enemy to the ageless athlete than doing too little, at least among highly motivated people. Consistently pushing too hard is what will lead to overtraining, overuse problems, and major injuries. If we are going to persist for decades, then at some level we need to moderate our instinctual desire to go hard.

We considered this problem at a "macro level" earlier, i.e., how to program for mandatory back-off days and even weeks in your training plan. Rest periods between workouts and blocks are important guards against doing too much, but equally crucial is guarding against doing too much within a single workout. In other words, you need to be able to make good **intra-workout decisions** about your load, intensity, volume, duration, etc., and this is particularly important for the middle-aged trainee who can't easily afford the consequences of a poor decision.

The problem, however, is that when you are having that great day and feeling that PR just around the corner, you're usually not in the best position to make a clear judgment. You are probably pumping with adrenaline. You might have a partner egging you on. There is just the spirit of the moment. It might be the day to push, but it will be hard to make a clear-headed judgment when you are in the middle of your seventeenth lap of Apex Hill Sprints. Get it right, and you get a great new notch in your belt. Get it wrong, and you can be set back for months. Here are some tips I have developed over the years to mitigate dumb intra-workout decision making.

Self-knowledge. Know your own temptations and potential psychological pitfalls. I love my kettlebell swings, and I take great pride in them. Thus, I have to mistrust myself when it comes to deciding whether I have had enough swings for the day. Thus, whenever I am tempted to really push the swing volume or add a few more laps than planned on Apex, I know that I need to take a second look and work extra hard to make a decision objectively. I have some real potential for costly self-deception in that vicinity. For me, the same attitude is necessary for long distance running. There is a nothing wrong with taking a 30-60 second break to clear your head for a moment and assess your status when you are thinking straight. Your personal weaknesses might be different from mine. You need to figure that out for yourself and remain vigilant. When you know that you are facing one of your perennial temptations to overdo it, be all the more cautious.

Planned Limits. It is probably a good idea to begin your workout with planned limits on how much you are willing to do. "Come what may, I'm only going to do X many sets of squats." This is something I do for my Apex sessions. Most days I will leave with the planned limit of fifteen rounds, no matter how good I am feeling. If I have an easy week coming or my other training has been light, I might lift the limit, but I need to be able to give myself a good reason. You can always ignore your own rules, but having a planned limit for the day makes it just a little harder psychologically to go too far. That small deterrence might make the difference.

Wise Training Partners. Intra-workout decision making can be particularly problematic when you train with other people. Training partners tend to push you harder, and that is part of what you want out of that relationship. That encouragement, however, can go too far. Good training partners should want you to get the best out of your training, and that also means knowing when to tell you to back off. Find people to train with who will hold you to high standards without pushing you to reckless extremes. Don't be afraid to separate yourself from training environments that hamper your real progress with too much "bro" bravado. I would rather still be going strong ten years from now than to be a "gym hero" today.

Get It Out of Your System. Give yourself some days to have all the fun you want (within the limits of reason!). Just as your diet will go better with the occasional cheat meal, you should every now and again indulge in an all-out training session. Just be smart about it. When I did my Duku-Duku challenge, I was in the middle of two-week deload. I had lots of rest going in and another full week to recover. I set an absolute limit of five rounds (which I barely completed), and I had someone on hand (my wife) whom I knew could be trusted "to pull the plug" if it looked like I'd had enough. It's fine to have some fun. Just don't throw everything away on one workout.

COMPETITION

There are a lot very good reasons to train for a formal competition, especially for an ageless athlete. Taking the risk to compete in a sport you have trained for over the course of months or years take guts. You have no idea how all that training will stack up until you "get into the ring," and there are no guaranteed outcomes in any competition. I don't care if it's a marathon, MMA bout, powerlifting meet, or a 5K race. Stepping into the arena against other people moves you from fantasy to reality, and it guards your fitness program against becoming a part of the narcissistic fantasies of a pathetic midlife crisis. Win or lose, you have done something for real. You will learn something positive about yourself: **I have the guts to stand up in front of other people and say "I can do this!"** Right now, I only compete in sports that I'm not terribly good at (running, triathlons, and BJJ), but I find those competitions to be the most fulfilling experiences in my greater than thirty-five year athletic history. Competing in situations wherein I feel honored just to be on the road or the mat with the people I'm facing stretches me to get better, grounds me in the real world, and keeps my ego in check. I urge you to find an arena of competition that does the same thing for you. Of course, I hope to win more in the future, too!

Furthermore, having a public deadline and putting some money down on an entry fee is not the worst motivator. Training simply to be "in shape" probably feels like building the proverbial bridge to nowhere. Without something you want to become good at and a clock ticking on how long you have to get there, it will at times be hard to answer the "What is the point?" question that will inevitably arise. One of the first questions I ask my clients who come to me for help with Tactical Barbell programming is, "What is something you want to use this program to become good at?" Don't just spin your wheels "working out," but instead train for mastery of an athletic craft.

More to our current point, however, is the fact that training for a competition is going to help you moderate some of your workouts. If I know I'm running a triathlon in two weeks, I'm going to be very disinclined not to push my hill sprints too hard and blow my Achilles tendon today. Pardon the pun, but with a competitive race around the corner, that's not the hill I want to die on. Likewise, if there is an impending BJJ tournament, I'm going to try very hard not to fry my CNS deadlifting. When you have something greater you are working for than just being the most impressive "worker-outer" at your local gym, you put every workout into its proper perspective. This or that workout is not the measure of me; it's only a means to the real test that I am working toward. By competing, you don't need to prove yourself in your workouts. That will happen on race day! It's better to impress fellow competitors at your next tournament than the crowd at your gym.

I try to schedule two or three fairly major (for me) competitions every year (BJJ tournaments, triathlons, road races). That keeps me grounded in reality and keeps my day-to-day workouts in proper perspective. If you are an operational athlete, you probably have plenty of things to keep you grounded in the real world and motivated to train. For civilians like me, the occasional competition is likely essential for ageless staying power.

CENTRAL TAKE-AWAYS FROM CHAPTER 18

- Use **self-knowledge**, **planned limits**, **wise training partners**, and the **occasional all-out effort** to support good intra-workout decision making.

- **Competition** is not only worthwhile in its own right, but supports good intra-workout decision making by giving you **goals that go beyond just intense workouts.**

CONCLUDING THOUGHTS

Chris Haueter, a renowned BJJ practioner and teacher, once said something to the effect that you are going to get ten years older, but the question is whether in the meantime you will earn a black belt. There is a lot of wisdom in this remark (and much else that Haueter has to say). The fact is that we are going to age. There is no doubt about that, and it's beyond our control. It's not up to any of us whether ten years will pass by. "Will I get old?" is a silly question, because the answer is a given. It's the human condition. How you age and what you will achieve along the way is another matter. What do you hope to have achieved during the next decade? That question is meaningful, because its answer is largely within your control. It is foolish to fret over the inevitable, whereas it is wise to plan for what is within your grasp.

Thus, I leave you with this question: **What do you want out of the next ten years of your life?** Whatever answer you give to that question, those ten years are going to come and go. Make your peace with that fact, and focus on what is within your power to change. How do you want to spend those ten years? Where do you want to be on the other side of the next decade?

Among those things that you can control over the next decade is your physical fitness. You will (hopefully!) be ten years older, but will you be in better shape than you are now? Will you be in the best shape of your entire life? I hope that this book has done something to help you see that affirmative answers to both of those questions are available to you whatever age you currently are, and there are definite steps you can take to make that happen. Now it is on you to execute.

I am rooting for you. If I can be any help along your journey, please reach out to me at the tacticalbarbell.com forum. I am also available for online coaching on an individual basis. Feel free to contact me at jim@tacticalbarbell.com.

NOTES

1 Plato, *Republic*, Book III, translated by G.M.A. Grube (Hackett, 1992).

2 See Pavel Tsatsouline, *Enter the Kettlebell: The Strength Secret of the Soviet Supermen* (Dragondoor, 2006).

3 K. Black, *Tactical Barbell: Definitive Strength Training for the Operational Athlete, Third Edition* (Zulu23 Group: 2016 – Print Edition); and *Tactical Barbell II: Conditioning* (K. Black: 2016 – Print Edition). All subsequent references to these texts are to the print editions.

4 David Mack and Gary Casstevens, *Mind Gym: An Athlete's Guide to Inner Excellence* (McGraw-Hill, 2002), p. 11.

5 For this and more about Lalanne's lifelong fitness achievements see http://jacklalanne.com/feats/ (accessed 12/26/16).

6 For the classic demonstration of the fundamental attribution error, see E.E. Jones and V.A. Harris, "The Attribution of Attitudes," *Journal of Experimental Social Psychology*, 1967, 3 (1): 1–24.

7 For the classic demonstration of self-serving bias, see J. Larson; U. Rutger; and C. Douglass, "Evidence for a Self-serving Bias in the Attribution of Causality," *Journal of Personality*, 1971, 45 (3): 430–441.

8 The information on Wildman was paraphrased from http://www.esquire.com/news-politics/a4454/don-wildman-0508/ (accessed 12/26/16) and http://www.latimes.com/health/la-he-0622-wildman-pictures-photogallery.html (accessed 12/26/16).

9 Seneca, *Moral Epistles*, translated by Richard M. Gummere (The Loeb Classical Library: 1917-25), quoted from stoics.com: http://www.stoics.com/seneca_epistles_book_1.html#%91XV1 (accessed 1/7/17).

10 K. Black, "How to be an Operational Athlete, Pt. 1," http://www.tacticalbarbell.

com/how-to-be-an-operational-athlete-part-1/ (accessed, 12/16/16). The following discussion of the concept of "operational athlete" is derived from this article and *Tactical Barbell*, pp. 23-24.

11 Aristotle, *Nicomachean Ethics*, Book II, Chapter 6.

12 See, C.J. Gochter and A. Baraki, "Heavy Lifting and Heart Health," http://startingstrength.com/contentfiles/heavy_lifting_heart.pdf (accessed 12/17/16); J.M. Sullivan and A. Baker, *The Barbell Prescription: Strength Training for Life After 40* (The Aasgaard Company, 2016); and references discussed at the beginning of chapter 5 of this volume.

13 For more on the Black protocol, see *Tactical Barbell II*, pp. 40-49.

14 Aristotle, *Nicomachean Ethics*, translated by W.D. Ross: http://classics.mit.edu/Aristotle/nicomachaen.2.ii.html (accessed 1/7/17).

15 L. Kilgore, M. Hartman, and J. Lascek, *Fit* (Killustrated, 2011), pp. 25-28.

16 Ibid., p. 25.

17 Pavel Tsatsouline, "Another Russian Super Cycle: Add up to 100 Pounds to Your Squat in Thirteen Weeks," http://www.dragondoor.com/articles/another-russian-super-cycle/ (accessed 12/18/16).

18 Pavel Tsatsouline, *Beyond Bodybuilding: Muscle and Strength Secrets for the Renaissance Man* (Dragondoor, 2005), pp. 23-24.

19 There is also a third, lower frequency template primarily intended for highly specialized athletes (MMA, boxing, BJJ, marathoners, triathletes, etc.) and military professionals who need to keep strength as a slightly lower priority compared to endurance and/or skills work year-round. For more information on the Fighter template, see *Tactical Barbell 3rd Ed.*, pp. 75-82.

20 For a detailed presentation of Operator, see ibid., pp. 47-55.

21 For a detailed presentation of Zulu, see ibid., pp. 65-69. I have introduced the Zulu I/A instead of Standard Zulu for the purposes of the comparative analysis of Operator and Zulu that follows below.

22 For a detailed presentation of Operator I/A, see ibid., pp. 56-61.

23 See *Tactical Barbell 3rd Edition*, pp. 83-86.

24 For explanations of these conditioning drills, see ibid., pp. 81-128.

25 The best program available focused on the mastering the swing is Pavel's *Simple and Sinister* (Strong First, Inc., 2013).

26 See Aristotle, *Nicomachean Ethics*, Book III, Chapters 6-9. For a very interesting

analysis of ancient Greek philosophers' views on physical training, see I. Theodoros, K. Marija, and

S. Đorđe, "Syncretism Of Coaching Science In Ancient Greece And Modern Times," *Serbian Journal of Sports Sciences*, 2008 (4), http://sjss-sportsacademy.edu.rs/archive/details/syncretism-of-coaching-science-in-ancient-greece-and-modern-times-35.html (accessed 12/26/16).

27 For a very accessible discussion of the physiological reasons why a solid sleep schedule is important to recovery, performance, and simple overall health, see Chapter IV of C. Hardy and M. Gallagher, *Strong Medicine: How to Conquer Chronic Disease and Achieve Your Full Genetic Potential* (Dragon Door Publications: 2015).

28 See Jim Wendler, *5/3/1: The Simplest and Most Effective Training System for Raw Strength*, 2nd Edition (Jim Wendler, LLC: 2011).

29 For a discussion of how to go about conducting a rep max test, see *Tactical Barbell 3rd Ed.*, pp. 87-90.

30 See *Tactical Barbell 3rd Ed.*, pp. 89-90.

31 Epictetus, *Enchiridion*, Chapter 29, in Epictetus, *Discourses and Selected Writings*, translated by Robert Dobbins (New York: Penguin Books, 2008), p. 233.

32 For a detailed case for including aerobic endurance training in the operational athlete's program, see *Tactical Barbell II*, pp. 17-27.

33 See ibid., pp. 35-37.

34 See ibid., pp. 38-39

35 For details on Tango, Alpha, and Bravo strength endurance circuits, see *Tactical Barbell 3rd Edition*, pp. 101-111.

36 *Tactical Barbell II*, pp. 35-37.

37 *Tactical Barbell 3rd Edition*, pp. 104-105.

38 By the way, the social psychologist who taught me about attribution error and self-serving biases is Jennifer L. Madden, Ph.D.

39 "9 Athletes over 60 Who Can Kick Your Butt," http://dailyburn.com/life/fitness/best-athletes-over-60/ (accessed 12/28/16).

40 Epictetus, *Discourses*, Book II, Chapter 18, in *Discourses and Selected Writings*.

41 There is some empirical evidence supporting what every gym rat has observed anecdotally: R. Rhodes RE and G. Bruij, "How Big is the Physical Activity Intention-behaviour Gap? A meta-analysis Using the Action Control Framework,"

British Journal of Health Psychology, 18 (2): 296-309. See also, http://www.bodybuilding.com/fun/2013-100k-transformation-contest-press-release.html (accessed 12/28/16).

42 If you are tempted to try a daily squatting program, tread carefully. You need to start slowly and be very patient. For more information, check out Matt Perryman's articles on this topic: https://www.myosynthesis.com/guide#daily-squats (accessed 12/28/16).

43 Aristotle, *Nicomachean Ethics*, translated by W.D. Ross: http://classics.mit.edu/Aristotle/nicomachaen.2.ii.html (accessed 1/7/17).

44 The idea that habituation is the primary means of building good character traits is not only the stuff of ancient philosophers. For empirical psychologists who defend this view, see M.E.P. Seligman, *Authentic Happiness* (New York: Free Press, 2002); and John Haidt, *The Happiness Hypothesis: Finding Modern Truth in Ancient Wisdom* (New York: Basic Books, 2006).

45 As of this writing "Sean" is just about to begin BUDS.